THE ANTIBODIES
Volume 7

THE ANTIBODIES
Volume 7

Edited by

Maurizio Zanetti, MD

*University of California
San Diego*

and

J. Donald Capra, MD

*Oklahoma Medical Research Foundation
Oklahoma City*

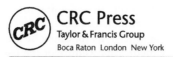

CRC Press
Taylor & Francis Group
Boca Raton London New York

CRC Press is an imprint of the
Taylor & Francis Group, an **informa** business

A TAYLOR & FRANCIS BOOK

First published 2002 by Taylor & Francis

Published 2019 by CRC Press
Taylor & Francis Group
6000 Broken Sound Parkway NW, Suite 300
Boca Raton, FL 33487-2742

© 2002 by Taylor & Francis Group, LLC
CRC Press is an imprint of Taylor & Francis Group, an Informa business

First issued in papaerback 2019

No claim to original U.S. Government works

ISBN 13: 978-0-367-45487-6 (pbk)
ISBN 13: 978-0-415-28466-0 (hbk)

Visit the Taylor & Francis Web site at
http://www.taylorandfrancis.com

and the CRC Press Web site at
http://www.crcpress.com

Typeset in Palatino by
Integra Software Services Pvt. Ltd, Pondicherry, India

Every effort has been made to ensure that the advice and information in this book is true and accurate at the time of going to press. However, neither the publisher nor the authors can accept any legal responsibility or liability for any errors or omissions that may be made. In the case of drug administration, any medical procedure or the use of technical equipment mentioned within this book, you are strongly advised to consult the manufacturer's guidelines.

British Library Cataloguing in Publication Data
A catalogue record for this book is available from the British Library

Library of Congress Cataloging in Publication Data
A catalog record for this book has been requested

CONTENTS

CONTENTS

SERIES PREFACE

Immunology is a discipline just over a century old that has played a central role in medicine and, more recently, in the biomedical sciences. Immunology has often been referred to as "imperialistic" for its tendency to spread to other biomedical fields like no other discipline. A myriad of publications have continually documented the incredible series of discoveries in this field. During times when many areas of immunology have undergone a formidable revolution, antibodies have always been central to any major progress in the field. From the pioneering work of von Behring and Kisatato at the end of the last century through the seminal experiments of Bordet, Ehrlich, Landsteiner, Oudin and Kunkel, just to name a few, and the conceptualizations of Burnet and Jerne, antibodies have dominated the scene. During the last two decades such major breakthroughs as the advent of monoclonal antibodies and the development of new techniques of antibody engineering have kept antibodies in the forefront of immunology and medical science. From diagnostic tools to vehicles for modern therapy against cancer, infections and autoimmune diseases, the study of antibodies has attracted a multitude of scientists.

While the race for better molecules for diagnosis and therapy is still on, it is evident that our knowledge of antibodies – their properties and structural characteristics – is still incomplete. Antibody genes and their regulation, intracellular assembly and secretion, antigen binding properties, effector function and immunity represent just a few of the topics that continue to be investigated using the tools of molecular biology, cell biology, immunochemistry, X-ray crystallography and computer-aided three-dimensional modeling. New technological developments now afford exploration of new areas of study and medical application for antibodies.

With *The Antibodies*, it is our intent to provide the scientific community with its first platform for a comprehensive review of topics of contemporary interest for specialists in this area. At the same time, we will take the opportunity to revisit more traditional aspects of the field so that relevant information and concepts are maintained in parallel with the more modern aspects. While the work ahead can be viewed with a sense of optimism and excitement, we do not underestimate the task that it will take to cover all areas of interest.

We extend our gratitude and thanks to all our colleagues who accepted our invitation to contribute their views and work, and who have made this volume a reality. We hope this collective effort will continue, contributing to keeping the field alive and exciting, and finding a legitimate identity in the immunological literature.

Maurizio Zanetti, MD
University of California
San Diego

J. Donald Capra, MD
Oklahoma Medical
Research Foundation
Oklahoma City

PREFACE

Volume 7

When this series began in 1995, we the editors intended to create a platform for updated information to specifically address issues relevant to the antibody molecule, Ig genes and the B-lymphocyte. We feel we have maintained our commitment with past volumes and see this continuing in Volume 7. The group of papers included in this volume cover aspects dealing more directly with (a) the genetic engineering of antibodies and their possible application; (b) the gene utilization and structure of anti-carbohydrates antibodies; and (c) some fundamental issues concerning the evolution of the V–D–J junctional region as well as the evolutionary necessity for a network of Ig V regions. We are pleased that Volume 7 covers such diverse topics and are certain that this collection of papers will once more put in perspective the field in its multi-faceted dimension.

In Chapter 1, Jacques Urbain and his colleagues revisit the concept of idiotypic networks starting with the provocative statement, "will idiotypic networks enjoy a vivid revival like suppressor T-cells?" This chapter redraws the parameters for a physiological role of the idiotypic network, focusing on its role in maintaining and shaping the repertoire of the newborn immune system. The authors argue that the major function of the idiotypic network is to induce transgenerational regulation and defenses at the level of adaptive immunity and that more generally idiotypic networks are used in building and shaping pre-memory B-cell lineages or "memories of the future." In assessing the value of neonatal idiotypic networks in ontogeny and phylogeny, the chapter restates in a forceful way that the immune system isn't merely a military machine designed to cope with the arrival of foreign invaders. Instead, through the idiotypic networks the immune system establishes not only its own survival, but also its own internal regulation and function independently of antigen. Based on selected experimental examples, the authors make a compelling argument in support of the fact that idiotype expression is governed mainly by the Igh locus and that anergic B-lymphocytes are in fact regulatory in shaping the immune repertoire through idiotypic complementarity.

In Chapter 2, Andrew Lew and his colleagues cover a new and exciting application for Ig genes in the design of more effective vaccines. By way of experimental examples, the chapter demonstrates that Ig molecules fused with ligands such as L-selectin or CTLA4 can direct the immunogenic process *in vivo* to the site of immune induction (lymph nodes and spleen) through selective binding to CD34 in high endothelial venules and CD80/CD86 on antigen presenting *cells*, respectively. This is a conceptually new way to use Ig fusion genes to deliver immunity effectively. The chapter describes in a succinct and incisive way recent accomplishments using these fusion genes, placing them in the context of the wider DNA vaccine field.

In Chapter 3, Harry Schroeder and his colleagues put Ig genes (V–D–J) under the microscope of evolution to identify patterns of amino acid expression in the heavy chain CDR3 (HCDR3) in mature B-cell repertoires. The chapter discusses the role of hydropathicity in selecting HCDR3 noting the existence of a pattern of similar hydropathicity among human, mouse and shark HCDR3s in spite of the fact that these three species are highly divergent, and trace their evolution in remarkably different environments. The author makes a compelling argument that the common pattern is based on a preference for neutral or slightly hydrophylic HCDR3 sequences. The significance of this finding is discussed in the context of the evolutionary advantage for the species, its survival, and the role in shaping the mature B-cell repertoire through recombination events.

In Chapter 4, Kathryn E. Stein and her colleagues revisit eloquently the nature and genetics of antibody responses against polysaccharides. Since these are constituents of the cell wall of bacteria, capsular factors and endotoxins, anti-polysaccharide responses occupy an important place in host-defense mechanisms. In a well organized tour de force, the chapter revisits the nature of anti-polysaccharide responses, and Igh gene usage against environmental, capsular and cell surface polysaccharides. This detailed and valuable up-to-date overview of the field ends with information on the structure of prototype anti-polysaccharide antibodies obtained by X-ray crystallography analysis. The chapter provides the reader with a modern appraisal of the nature, genetics and three-dimensional structure of anti-polysaccharide antibodies.

In Chapter 5, Rainer Fischer and colleagues offer a complete and well-documented overview of the current art in antibody farming, i.e., the production of antibodies in plants that can be cultivated on an agricultural scale. While the science of antibody farming began only a decade ago, much progress has been made since due to the important pharmaceutical and economical implications.

This chapter covers in detail the basic premises to antibody engineering and phage-display technology for the generation of combinatorial library after *in vivo* immunization or *in vitro* selection. It also provides insights into approaches to select for given specificities and improve antibody affinity. As to expression systems, the chapter describes clearly the path to produce antibodies by plant farming. The reader will also find information on transgenic plants and insights on how transgenesis with antibody genes may lead to improving crops with disease resistance genes. Finally, the chapter covers initial therapeutic applications of plant-derived antibodies with special emphasis on IgA antibodies and results of clinical trials using plant-derived antibodies. The reader will no doubt see that this chapter constitutes a state-of-the-art review and analysis of antibody engineering applied to plant expression systems.

Maurizio Zanetti, MD   *J. Donald Capra, MD*
University of California   Oklahoma Medical
San Diego   Research Foundation
                                                 Oklahoma City

CONTRIBUTORS

Olga Artsaenko, Institut für Biologie I, Aachen, Germany

Jeffrey S. Boyle, CSL Ltd, Parkville, Australia

Jamie L. Brady, The Walter & Eliza Hall Institute of Medical Research, Parkville, Australia

Maryse Brait, Université Libre de Bruxelles, Gosselies, Belgium

Kurt Brorson, Center for Biologics Evaluation and Research, Bethesda, USA

Alexandra J. Corbett, The Walter & Eliza Hall Institute of Medical Research, Parkville, Australia

Carl De Trez, Université Libre de Bruxelles, Gosselies, Belgium

Ricarda Finnern, Institut für Biologie I, Aachen, Germany

Rainer Fischer, Institut für Biologie I, Aachen, Germany and Fraunhofer Abteilung für Molekulare Biotechnologie, Schmallenberg, Germany

Pablo Garcia-Ojeda, Center for Biologics Evaluation and Research, Bethesda, USA

Gregory C. Ippolito, University of Alabama at Birmingham, USA

Ivaylo Ivanov, University of Alabama at Birmingham, USA

Stephen J. Kent, University of Melbourne, Australia

David R. Kramer, Deakin University, Burwood, Australia

Oberdan Leo, Université Libre de Bruxelles, Gosselies, Belgium

Andrew M. Lew, The Walter & Eliza Hall Institute of Medical Research, Parkville, Australia

Jason Link, University of Alabama at Birmingham, USA

Chantal Masungi Luko, Université Libre de Bruxelles, Gosselies, Belgium

Brent S. McKenzie, The Walter & Eliza Hall Institute of Medical Research, Parkville, Australia

Robert Miller, University of New Mexico, Albuquerque, USA

Martin J. Pearse, CSL Ltd, Parkville, Australia

Roy Riblet, Torry Pines Institute of Molecular Studies, San Diego, USA

Stefan Schillberg, Institut für Biologie I, Aachen, Germany

Harry W. Schroeder, Jr., University of Alabama at Birmingham, USA

Kathryn E. Stein, Center for Biologics Evaluation and Research, Bethesda, USA

Richard A. Strugnell, University of Melbourne, Australia

Robyn M. Sutherland, The Walter & Eliza Hall Institute of Medical Research, Parkville, Australia

Jacques Urbain, Université Libre de Bruxelles, Gosselies, Belgium

Annette Van Acker, Université Libre de Bruxelles, Gosselies, Belgium

Georgette Vansanten, Université Libre de Bruxelles, Gosselies, Belgium

Christian Wuilmart, Université Libre de Bruxelles, Gosselies, Belgium

Chapter

ONE

Positive Selection of B-Cell Repertoire, Idiotype Networks and Immunological Memory

Maryse Brait[1], Georgette Vansanten[1], Annette Van Acker[1], Carl De Trez[1], Chantal Masungi Luko[1], Christian Wuilmart[1], Oberdan Leo[1], Robert Miller[2], Roy Riblet[3], and Jacques Urbain[1]

[1]*Laboratory of Animal Physiology, Institute of Molecular Biology and Medicine (IBMM), Université Libre de Bruxelles, 12, Rue des Professeurs Jeener et Brachet, 6041 Gosselies, Belgium*
[2]*University of New Mexico, Department of Biology, 288 Castetter Hall, Albuquerque 87131-1091, USA*
[3]*Torrey Pines Inst. Molec.Studies, 3550 General Atomics Court, San Diego CA 92121, USA*

I. INTRODUCTION

Idiotype network theories became very popular in the early 1970s. Numerous papers have been devoted to networks, but after a glory period, network theories were nearly forgotten and fell into the same disgrace as suppressor T-cells [1] (except that suppressor T-cells are now enjoying a vivid revival [2]). Even today, papers which claim that V regions of Ig receptors on naïve B-lymphocytes are essential for lymphocyte survival, ignore idiotype network ideas [3]. It has been said that idiotype networks are just a footnote in the history of immunology [4].

Address correspondence to: Jacques Urbain, Laboratory of Animal Physiology, Institute of Molecular Biology and Medicine (IBMM), Université Libre de Bruxelles, 12, Rue des Professeurs Jeener et Brachet, 6041 Gosselies, Belgium. e-mail: jurbain@dbm.ulb.ac.be and jaurbain@ulb.ac.be

As noted by M. Cohn [5]: "Today the tide of regulation via idiotype networks has receded behind an empty beach...and we have no idea what it was that produced the tidal wave or its ebb. If we find ourselves asking 'Whatever happened to... ?', it is safe to say that we never learned anything from it."

The concepts of idiotype networks have been removed from recent texbooks. So it was a pleasant surprise to read the following in a recent paper of C.A. Janeway [6]: "Jerne's idiotypic network actually can act on the naïve B-cell repertoire to positively select certain heavy/light chain pairs over others." This is exactly what was proposed by A. Coutinho and ourselves, among others, many years ago [7–9]. Will idiotypic networks enjoy a vivid revival like suppressor T-cells?

Even if some criticisms against network theories were right–the network theory was unable to cope with several important regulatory mechanisms in the immune system, i.e., the self–non-self discrimination phenomenon and the regulation of class effectors (11)–it is unfair to conclude that nothing was learned from a study of the concept.

In fact, we see three major reasons for the importance of idiotype networks:

1   An idiotype network can help explain the maintenance of a vast array of V, D...gene segments during evolution.
2   It is difficult (or almost impossible) to interpret "idiotype imprinting à la Konrad Lorenz" without idiotype networks (see the excellent review by Lemke and Lange [12]).
3   The idiotype priming by maternal effects implies positive idiotypic B-cell selection during ontogeny, and recent data seem to establish such a positive selection (see below).

This paper deals mainly with points 2 and 3. We shall only comment briefly on point 1, which in fact brings some authors of this paper to propose idiotype network concepts. A complete variable region gene is a somatic construct of V_H, D_H, and J_H elements brought together by DNA rearrangements in B-cells. Two hypervariable regions are located within the V gene segment. The fully assembled third CDR, which spans the joint of a VDJ rearrangement, is not found in higher vertebrates, and this third hypervariable region seems to be the most important for antigen binding. How do we explain the presence of highly non-random patterns in the germline V gene DNA which can only arise by direct antigen-binding selection forces acting on the gene product and not the DNA directly? How can we maintain the Wu-Kabat signature at the level of the germline even if most antigens will not be encountered during the lifetime of one individual? Steele *et al.* [13] have proposed a Lamarckian explanation (transfer of DNA from soma to germline; i.e., transfer of DNA from mutated B-lymphocytes to germ cells) for that paradox and have written an entire book on the subject. A more conservative explanation for the Wu-Kabat structure of germline genes is to suppose that many mutations in the CDR are neutral or advantageous while most mutations in framework regions lead mainly to non-functional antibodies. This conventional evolution can probably be much faster and more efficient if there is a functional idiotype network during ontogeny providing an internal selective pressure in the absence of foreign antigens [14, 15]. This kind of evolution will reinforce connectivity and could be a partial explanation for the high connectivity of the pre-immune repertoire together with a preferential loss of unconnected idiotypes.

(A detailed evolutionary scheme will be presented elsewhere.) This in turn implies idiotype maternal imprinting, which requires positive selection of B-lymphocytes by internal idiotypic cascades.

Several experimental facts, repeatedly established in several experimental models and different species, argue strongly that the immune system can behave as an idiotype network in physiological experiments [16, 17]. More precisely, the so-called idiotype mimicry phenomena – i.e., the presence of a given maternal idiotype convinces the lymphocytes of the newborn to make the same or a very similar idiotype – imply that some idiotypes are endowed with regulatory power, which is precisely the crux of the network theory. It seems difficult to imagine a more physiological experiment than exposure of a fetal or neonatal immune system to maternal effects.

It has been proven beyond doubt that the results of some of these experiments cannot be explained by antigen or cell transfers from the mother to the fetus. In a way we could say that the baby acquires the immunological knowledge of the mother, which makes good sense in evolutionary terms.

In fact, it has been shown recently that this learning can also take place for non-adaptive defense mechanisms. For example, when Agrawal et al. [18] exposed water fleas to kairomones from two invertebrate predators, the water fleas developed long helmets. Furthermore, offspring of kairomone-treated mothers produced longer helmets than offspring from control mothers, in whatever environment offspring were raised. The authors saw the same effects in successive broods produced later by kairomone-treated mothers in clean water. Thus, development of long helmets in embryonic stages resulted from maternal effects and did not need to be induced directly by the chemical cues called kairomones. Induced defenses can extend across generations. Similar observations were made in plant defenses. Transgenerational induction of defenses are a new level of phenotypic plasticity across generations that may be an important component of predator–prey interactions.

In this paper we shall argue that the major function of the idiotype network is to induce transgenerational defenses at the level of adaptive immunity and that more generally, idiotype networks are used in building and shaping of what we have called "memories of the future" or the "pre-memory B-cell lineage."

The role of maternal protection should not be underestimated. It should be emphasized that the concept of immunological memory remains an enigma. As stated by R. Zinkernagel [19]: "Why should the host need memory? If the host survives the first infection, the host immune system has proven itself fit to deal with repeat infections; if the host is killed by the first infection there is no need of immunological memory. Under such circumstances, is immunological memory of survival value? The main role of memory is to overcome problems of infectious diseases during the time needed for maturation of the newborn immune system. This is dramatically illustrated by the fact that most calves not given colostral milk during the first 18 hours after birth – the short period when intact antibodies can be absorbed in the gut – do not possess protective maternal antibodies and die of infections within weeks."

This maternal protection is essential for species survival, and we shall argue the idiotype network can prime the newborn immune according to maternal experience. This idiotypic priming implies, of course, a positive selection of some

B-lymphocytes, and we shall propose that this positive selection plays a major role in the generation of immunological memory partly due to internal idiotype cascades.

II. FORMAL NETWORKS AND INTERNAL IMAGES

The immune system is able to respond to an enormous array of antigenic struc- tures. But every idiotype can also induce the synthesis of anti-idiotypic antibodies. These two sets of antibodies must be largely overlapping. In other words, the diversity of the immune system is such that, as a statistical necessity, idiotypes and auto-anti-idiotypes coexist inside the repertoire of one individual. By the same token, auto-anti-idiotypes coexist with anti-anti-idiotypes. The immune sys- tem forms a web of V domains and cannot avoid the recognition of itself. This has been called the formal network which, in a simplified manner, can be represented by a cascade Ag (+) $\rightarrow$ Ab1(−) $\rightarrow$ Ab2(+) $\rightarrow$ Ab3(−) $\rightarrow$ Ab4(+) . . .

In fact, such a cascade has been studied using different rabbits for each step of the cascade [20–22]. The bulk of Ab3 antibodies is made up of molecules sharing idiotypic specificities with Ab1, but are non-antigen binding. This set (the parallel set) is denoted id+ag−. A subpopulation of Ab3 antibodies shares idiotypic speci- ficities with Ab1, but in addition, binds antigen (id+ag+). This subset is selected and amplified after antigen immunization and gives rise to the so-called 'Ab1' subset of antibodies. In addition, part of Ab4 looks like Ab2 [23].

Inside the repertoire of one individual, the presence of complementary partners has been demonstrated repeatedly. The network hypothesis states this coexistence has regulatory consequences in the functioning of the immune system. The immune system is using its own diversity to regulate itself. As such the hypothesis is rather vague in the sense that it does not predict the regulatory con- sequences. The hypothesis predicts that the immune system has an inner life in the absence of foreign antigen. The immune system is not only a military machine designed to cope with the arrival of foreign invaders.

From the concept of formal networks emerges the concept of internal images. Let us consider an idiotype recognizing antigen X. This idiotype can also be rec- ognized by several anti-idiotypes; the diversity of the system is such that some anti-idiotypes could bear a "positive image" of the antigen, recognizing on the idiotype the same area of the active site as the one recognized by antigen. This does not imply the three-dimensional structure of the internal image is a perfect match of the antigenic determinant.

The concept of internal image received its first experimental support from the studies of Sege and Peterson [24, 25]. Rabbit anti-idiotypic antibodies were raised against rat anti-insulin-antibodies. These anti-idiotypic antibodies are able to inhibit the binding of insulin to raT-cells. These anti-idiotypic antibodies also bind to the insulin receptor and can mimic insulin.

Some rabbit anti-idiotypic antibodies to rabbit anti-TMV (tobacco mosaic virus) are clear examples of internal images [26]. Such anti-idiotypes react with anti- TMV antibodies from other rabbits, chickens, goats and horses. Furthermore, some rabbit anti-idiotypic antibodies injected into mice, which have never seen the virus induce anti-TMV antibodies [27], behave like antigen. Structural simi- larities have been found between anti-idiotypic antibodies and antigen, notably in the GAT system [28].

The crystal structure of an idiotype recognizing lyzozyme anti-idiotope complex has been determined. The anti-lyzozyme antibody uses essentially the same combining site to bind the lyzozyme or the anti-idiotope. Particularly striking is the fact that of the 18 residues used by the antibody to contact the anti-idiotope, 13 are also in contact with lyzozyme. In this particular case, the hypervariable regions of Ab2 which are not helical can "mimic" the structure of an epitope which is partly alpha helical [29]. As stated by the authors, the mimicking is functional, involving similar binding interactions rather than exact topological replicas, which in most cases would be almost impossible to achieve, especially for anti-idiotypic antibodies acting as surrogates of antigen which are not proteins (e.g., carbohydrates). Finally, these Ab2 antibodies have been shown to induce anti-lyzozyme antibodies.

Another interesting anti-idiotopic system is a large glycoprotein antigen, E2, from the feline infections peritonitis virus [30]. The complex formed by Fab fragments of Ab1 and Ab2 has been crystallized and the three-dimensional structure at 2.9 Å resolution has been determined. A comparison of sequences revealed a strong homology between two hexapeptides located in the CDR of Ab2 and the E2 antigen. In this case, the authors suggest a transmission of information through the anti-idiotopic by linear sequence preservation.

Also some recent examples using abzymes are particularly striking [31]. BALB/C mice were immunized with Bacillus β-lactamase. From 150 monoclonal antibodies, one was chosen to immunize, an MAb that significantly inhibited the enzyme. All antibodies induced were accompanied by a significant increase of β-lactamase activity. One isolated hybridoma from Ab2 was able to hydrolyze penicillinic and cephalosporinic substrates with Michaelis-Menten kinetics. So starting with an enzyme antigen, it is possible to obtain anti-idiotypic antibodies, which exhibit enzymatic properties.

As stated above, the idiotype network hypothesis rests on the assumption of the coexistence of complementary partners in the repertoire of one individual.

It was shown long ago that rabbits can make anti-idiotypic antibodies when injected with the idiotype previously synthesized by the same animal [32, 33].

Kluskens and Köhler [34] were the first to demonstrate the appearance of spontaneous auto-anti-idiotypic antibodies in BALB/C mice immunized with *Streptococcus pneumoniae*. Furthermore, this response is characterized by multiple waves of idiotypes and auto-anti-idiotypes. Spontaneous auto-anti-idiotypes have also been described in the response of rabbits to TMV [35].

Some auto-anti-idiotypic or syngeneic antibodies exhibit unusual properties. In mice, syngeneic auto-anti-idiotypic antibodies are notoriously difficult to induce. Lange and Lemke [36] used the 2-phenyloxazolone system (phOx) where the primary response is characterized by a dominant idiotype (idOx1) and is replaced by other idiotypes in the secondary and tertiary responses. As compared to the response to conventional antigen (including oxazolone), the anti-idiotypic response in syngeneic mice exhibits a lag phase of three weeks.

An anti-idiotypic antibody secondary response could be induced even with the soluble idiotype, but the level of the anti-idiotypic antibodies after boosting was not higher than in the primary response. During this secondary response, idiotypically non-related IgM anti-hapten antibodies appear. There is thus an intriguing dissymmetry between the idiotypic and anti-idiotypic response.

The frequency of auto-anti-idiotypic B-cells was investigated using the arsonate system in A/J mice by limiting dilution analysis after polyclonal activation with lipopolysaccharide (LPS) [37]. While the frequency of B-cells able to produce the idiotype is detectable in every naïve A/J mouse (the frequency is around 10^{-4}), the precursor frequencies of auto-Ab2 B-cells were below the limit of sensitivity of the technique in the majority of A/J mice. Auto-Ab2 B-cells could be detected in only 20% of naïve A/J mice. Upon immunization with Ars-KLH, however, a large increase in auto-Ab2 precursor frequency was found (10^3-fold). This effect was seen very early after immunization (six days). These results suggest the frequency of B-lymphocytes potentially able to produce auto-anti-idiotypic antibodies is much higher than the measured frequency. Significantly, this shift is not observed when A/J mice are injected with KLH or when BALB/C mice that do not produce the CRI_A idiotype are injected with Ars-KLH. As in the previous case, the auto-Ab2 lymphocytes are somewhat impaired in their activation properties.

Once again there is a striking dissymmetry between Ab1 and Ab2. Several explanations can be considered, either structural or physiological. One of them posits that in some idiotypic systems Ab1 and Ab2 precursors belong to distinct lymphocyte compartments or subsets and that Ab2 precursors belong to the subset of anergic or tolerant B-lymphocytes [35]. Such a state of anergy could be transiently broken by immunization, e.g., Ars-KLH in A/J mice by bringing auto-Ab2 precursors in the vicinity of helper T-cells. Structural explanations (such as rare V–D–J combination or rare N regions) cannot account for the observations.

III. THE NETWORK THEORY AND IDIOTYPE REGULATION

In his remarkable book, "A History of Immunology," A. Silverstein [38] explains how network theories go back to the side chain theory of Ehrlich. "*Perhaps the best known instance of a premature theory was Ehrlich side chain theory of 1897.*" This model was for all practical purposes, the first natural selection theory of antibody formation. It dominated the field for perhaps a decade, only to fall in disrepute and nearly be forgotten for half a century until Jerne and Burnet gave the selective theory of antibody formation its modern form and appeal. But Ehrlich's theory was more than the concept of antibody formation: it speculated broadly also (within the obvious limitations of contemporary scientific knowledge) about the structure and function of antibodies.

Implicit in the side chain theory was an even more startling conceptual anticipation of the future: the binding site of an antibody is a unique structure and might be immunogenic, an anti-antibody might be formed against the specific site, the shape of an anti-antibody combining site would be that of the corresponding antigen for which the original antibody was specific.

In 1967, Gell and Kelus [39] reviewed the literature about autoantibodies and idiotypes. With impressive foresight they wrote: "*It is hard to believe that the body can regularly react to private determinants on its own antibodies not so much because the process would be self-destructive as that it would lead to an infinite regress of anti-antibody production.*" Furthermore, they proposed that self-tolerance to idiotypic determinants, in the sense of clonal deletion, does not provide a likely explanation since, "*it would entail the elimination of a number of clones equal to the number of possible* antibodies." So they first realized the universe of potential anti-idiotypes might equal in size the universe of possible antibodies. This concept is the basis of Jerne's network theory summarized below [40, 41].

If we consider only the idiotypic properties of an antibody, an immunoglobulin can be described as p1-i1 where p1 is the active side (paratope) recognizing the epitope E and i1 is the set of idiotopes outside the paratope. Now p1 can also recognize the idiotopes i2 of a molecule p2-i2. I2 can therefore be called an internal image. On the molecule p1-i1, the set of idiotopes i1 recognize the paratope p3 of the anti-idiotopic set p3-i3 and so on. These p2-i2 and p3-i3 are thus anti-idiotypic molecules. As a crude approximation, Jerne proposed that recognition of paratopes on lymphocytes led to stimulation while recognition of idiotopes led to suppression. Therefore, any immune response is a perturbation of an internal equilibrium reached through activating and suppressive idiotypic interactions. Using this framework, Jerne tried to explain the low zone tolerance phenomenon, the 7S inhibition effect, the breaking of tolerance by crossreactive antigens, the antigenic competition phenomena, and the existence of parallel sets. Network concepts were also proposed on the basis of quite distinct premises. For example, Urbain [42] proposed a network concept to solve the problem of maintaining a large number of germline genes with their Wu-Kabat structure, i.e., germline genes in which the CDR can be easily identified without the need of somatic mutations and the selection of available repertoire.

Is the immune system a functional idiotype network? Is the network selfish with no obvious regulatory advantage? The mere fact an immune response can be obtained without idiotypic interactions is not proof of the absence of idiotypic regulation. The data obtained from idiotype manipulations (suppression or activation by anti-idiotypic antibodies, idiotype vaccines) do not need the existence of a functional network but can be explained in terms of clonal selection alone.

As an advent of immune receptor diversification and the almost limitless heterogeneity of the repertoire, a new problem arose in evolution. The immune system had to deal with connectivity creating a noisy background due to idiotypic interactions between V genes within the repertoire of a single individual. At a more basic level, such a problem had already been encountered and solved in the evolution of organisms. At first, genetic networks (interactions between the products of different genes or between the products and the genes) must lead to noise but also and mainly, to coherent regulatory circuits resistant to unavoidable noise.

It is highly unlikely that selection alone can extract order from chaos; rather self-organizing properties of networks must provide a partial solution towards meaningful regulation. Genetic redundancy, repression, and mainly hierarchical control of genes offer partial clues to reduce the noise of undesirable interactions.

Leaving aside T-cells whose receptors are mainly concerned with MHC molecules, we have proposed a model of the ontogeny of idiotype networks for B-lymphocytes [9]. The model predicts the presence of maternal or early Ab1 will promote the induction of Ab1 in the offspring. The new immune system can learn the historical experience of the mothers. It should be emphasized that the model was not designed to explain the effects of maternal immunity but was prompted by the relationships between immunological tolerance and idiotype networks.

We first must distinguish between the somatic self and the immunological self: the somatic self is the whole self minus V regions. The diversity of the somatic self and the immunological self differ by orders of magnitude. The immune system cannot become tolerant to all idiotypes because this will lead to an empty immune system.

As precursors of B-lymphocytes develop, some of them will be confronted with somatic self-antigen. There is considerable strong evidence from old and new data using transgenic mice that such B-lymphocytes will be rendered anergic (tolerant).

We then suppose such anergic B-lymphocytes are not simply condemned to death but will perform a regulatory function through idiotype interactions. More precisely, such regulatory B-lymphocytes will be responsible for positive selection of their complementary partners (i.e., auto Ab2 lymphocytes). As usual, positive selection means acquisition of a longer life span. B-lymphocytes with a long life span will tend to become dominant in immune responses against external antigens, i.e., some recurrent idiotypes are anti-idiotypes of antiself idiotypes. Idiotype dominance is then predicted by broken symmetries in the preimmune repertoire. Such anti-antiself idiotypes constitute the repertoire of the "prememory B-cell pool," which could correspond to some extent to the HSA^{low} subset [43].

As unselected B-lymphocytes enter the primary B-cell pool (the HSA^{high} subset), there is nothing that can distinguish a self-epitope from a self-idiotope. Therefore, self-idiotopes present on maternal idiotypes can reach sufficient concentrations to be treated as self-epitopes. Therefore, maternal idiotype will tolerize anti-idiotypic B-cells which will positively select complementary partners (including Ab1). In this context, maternal Ab1 idiotypes can prime for offspring Ab1 idiotypes. By the same token, the presence of Ab2 can lead to long-term suppression of Ab1. At the level of T-cells, it has been shown that anergic T-cells can become regulatory T-cells [44].

The first example of idiotype mimicry was reported in a private idiotypic system using rabbits immunized against TMV. Irradiated recipients of a3 allotype (a marker of V regions) were repopulated with hyperimmune spleen or bone marrow cells from donors bearing the a1 allotype. Recipient rabbits, when immunized with TMV, produce antibodies idiotypically cross-reactive with donor antibodies despite the fact that different rabbits immunized against TMV produce antibodies idiotypically non-crossreactive. The use of the a allotype marker establishes the fact that recipient antibodies were indeed synthesized by recipienT-cells and not by donor cells. This was interpreted to suggest that the presence of donor cells had idiotypically imprinted the emerging immune system from the irradiated recipients [45].

The same conclusions can be reached by considering the results of maternal effects in the *Micrococcus lysodeikticus* antigenic system – for example, the case of female rabbits learning to synthesize a silent idiotype by the idiotypic cascade [46]. These female rabbits produce Ab3 antibodies. Only a very small subset of these Ab3 antibodies are able to bind antigen. These female rabbits, that have never been exposed to antigen, are crossed with naïve males. After two months, the mothers, fathers and offspring are injected with antigen. All synthesize large amounts of anti-carbohydrate antibodies but now *40% of the offspring make the same idiotype as the mothers*. It is evident in this system of idiotypes "à la Oudin" that the idiotype present in the offspring is really synthesized by the offspring. As expected, males synthesize unrelated idiotypes.

The level of Ab3 antibodies transmitted to the offspring is such that this Ab3 can be considered as a somatic self-antigen by the immune system of the neonate. Therefore, anti-Ab3 lymphocytes will be anergized and will positively select complementary partners (i.e., Ab3). When the offspring are confronted with antigen, the small population of Ab1' lymphocytes will be expanded. An early transient perturbation of the neonate has been integrated into long-term memory.

By the same token, it is easy to see that exposure of the neonate to Ab2 will predispose them to make Ab2, and this can explain long-term idiotype suppression of the neonate.

Also, it can be predicted that early antigen exposure or early anti-mu treatment will perturb positive selection and lead to the loss of idiotype dominance. The model also predicts removal of auto-anti-idiotypic B-cells in the early repertoire will impede selection of the pre-memory B-cell pool and will lead to the loss of idiotype dominance in some systems. Other experiments lead to the same conclusions.

Two recent studies are striking: Montesano et al. [47], and Lemke and Lange, [12]. Many studies on different human parasitic diseases have shown an effect of maternal infectious status on the immune response of the child. In addition, two field studies have shown these effects on the immune system can persist for up to 20 years. Upon infection, people born and raised in areas with a high prevalence of schistosomiasis generally develop only the intestinal form of chronic diseases with less than 10 per cent of individuals progressing to hepatosplenic disease. In contrast, travelers or recent immigrants to an endemic area often present acute illness if they become infected.

The authors have examined a possible role of maternal idiotypic interactions in Schistosoma mansoni infections using idiotypic manipulation of the neonatal immune system. Mice that received appropriate idiotype injections during the first 24 hours of life displayed altered immune responses, decreased pathology, and increased long-term survival upon infection with Schistosoma. In addition, mice injected with idiotype within the first day of birth have idiotype in their serum after eight weeks, even in the absence of subsequent infection or exposure to Schistosoma antigen. The idiotype levels far exceed the amount of initially injected idiotype. These results strongly suggest that neonatal idiotype injections induce animals to produce idiotype.

As described above, the early immune response of BALB/C mice immunized with 2-phenyloxazolone (phOX) is dominated by a recurrent idiotype named IdOx1. As the response proceeds, IdOx is replaced by other idiotypes. The tertiary and quaternary responses are practically devoid of the IdOx1 idiotype. Lange et al. [48] demonstrated that maternal tertiary immunization or quaternary antibodies induced dramatic alterations in the F1 and F2 primary repertoires. The proportion of the Ox1 idiotype is reduced in the majority of mice. More strikingly, the non IdOx1 showed a 5- to 100-fold enhanced affinity.

The non-IdOx1 were encoded by V_H and V_L gene combination unobserved in the anti-phOX response or typical of memory responses in normal mice. Thus maternal antibodies which are acquired during maturation may have an epigenetic (non-Mendelian) inheritable potential for the offspring.

All these studies demonstrate that maternal immunoglobulins do not just function as a passive protection device but initiate a cascade of events imprinting the neonate immune system for the rest of its life. It seems these facts cannot be explained by theories envisioning the antigen as the sole selective agent regulating the immune responses. Other examples of idiotype mimicry have been described in Forni *et al.* [49] and Martinez *et al.* [50].

IV. THE ARSONATE SYSTEM

Linkage to the Igh Locus

The response of A/J mice to arsonate hapten conjugated to a carrier protein like keyhole limped hemocyanin (Ars-KLH) is characterized by the synthesis of antibodies sharing intrastrain crossreactive idiotypic specificities (CRI). These antibodies were defined by polyclonal rabbit antisera to the anti-arsonate antibodies adsorbed with pre-immune A/J sera [51].

Hybridoma technology had a major impact for detailed analysis of the arsonate system. CRI-positive hybridoma antibodies have been classified in three distinct antibody families: Ars A, Ars B, and Ars C [51]. The Ars A antibody family is A/J strain specific. The Ars B and Ars C families are present in both A/J and BALB/C mice. The idiotypes associated with each family have been termed CRIA, CRIB, and CRIC. CRIC idiotype dominates the BALB/C anti-arsonate response. A few years later, another CRI idiotype was described and termed CRID. CRID antibodies are formed by the Ars A light chains and CRI C heavy chains [53].

The molecular basis of the CRIA has been extensively studied. The heavy chain is made up of one unique VH gene segment (VH IdCR11 belonging to J558 family), one D gene segment (DFL16.1), and one JH gene segment (JH2). The VK10.1 and JK1 gene segments encode the kappa light chain. This unique combination of gene segments has been termed the "Canonical Combination." Two specific junctional residues necessary for Ars binding have been characterized: serine at position 99 in the VHIdCR11-DFL16.1 junction [54] and arginine at position 96 in the VK-JK1 junction [55]. The primary anti-arsonate response is clonally diverse and CRIA antibodies constitute only a modest fraction of the response. Only near the end of the primary response and in the secondary response, CRIA antibodies become predominant. Molecular analysis has revealed that in the beginning of the anti-arsonate response, the VHIdCR11 segment is associated with a collection of different D, JH gene segments and kappa light chains. As the response proceeds, the canonical combination is selected and dominates. This unique combination of gene segments continues to dominate anamnestic responses. CRIA gene segments undergo extensive somatic hypermutation. Recurrent VH region amino acid substitutions due to somatic hypermutation have been identified. They confer increased affinity for arsonate hapten [55–59].

Different laboratories, including our own, have derived monoclonal anti-idiotypic antibodies to dissect the CRIA idiotype. Anti-idiotypic antibodies are given the same name as the target idiotope they recognize. Briefly, the mAb 7B7 derived in the Nisonoff laboratory is CRIA light chain specific. It recognizes amino acids in the second and third hypervariable regions. Our laboratory has isolated four mAb, namely 2D3, E4, E3 and H8. mAb detect the last three different idiotopes for which the expression is mainly dependent on the DFL16.1 gene segment. 2D3 mAb recognizes an idiotope located in the second hypervariable region of the VHIdCR11, more precisely 2D3 idiotope expression is linked to lysine 59. The detailed properties of these anti-idiotypic monoclonal antibodies are described in Leo *et al.* [60], Jeske *et al.* [61] and Hasemann and Capra [62].

Extensive breeding studies performed by Nisonoff's group initially restricted the CRIA antibody expression to the heavy chain loci Igh e (A/J) and o (AL/N) haplotypes. BALB/C mice are considered a CRIA negative strain [51]. Linkage to the Igh locus was shown by tests carried out with C.AL-20 congenic mice [63]. C.AL mice carry the Igh o locus of AL/N strain on a BALB/C background. In all these experiments, the anti-arsonate responses were analyzed with specific polyclonal antisera raised against A/J anti-arsonate antibodies and extensively adsorbed on pre-immune A/J immunoglobulins.

Later it was shown that the ability to express the CRIA idiotype was linked to both heavy and light chain loci [64, 65]. In genetic crosses, most strains could provide the appropriate light chain, but others (i.e., C58, AKR, PL/J) could not. The strains unable to complement the A strain heavy chain were reminiscent of studies showing polymorphism for kappa light chain phenotypic markers like IB [66, 67] and Ef1a isoelectrofocusing marker [68]. These two markers were due to polymorphism at the IgK-Vser locus [69, 70] now referred to as the IgK-V28 locus [71].

Studies at the DNA level firmly established a link between the CRIA antibody expression and the presence of the VHIdCR11 in the genome. BALB/C mice do not possess this particular gene segment and are consequently CRIA negative [72, 73]. The VK10 gene family with the VK10.1 member encoding for the CRIA light chain has been divided in two allelic groups by RFPL analysis among mouse strains [55, 74, 75]. One is the IgK V10a restricted to the strains presenting the polymorphism at the IgK V28 locus (AKR, C58 . . .). The other allele is the IGK V10b found in most mouse strains (A/J, BALB/C . . .). The product of the AKR IgK V10.1a gene segment contained four amino acid substitutions in the CDR3 as compared with the CRIA IgK V10.1b product. These substitutions explain the failure of AKR mice and the other strains with the same VK10 RFLP pattern to provide an appropriate light chain to form CRIA antibodies in genetic crosses.

At first sight, molecular studies lead to a simple situation: CRIA idiotype expression is correlated with the presence of the right VH and VK gene segments in the genome.

Using anti-idiotypic monoclonal antibodies, we have also performed analysis of anti-arsonate responses of new heavy chain allotype congenic between A/J and BALB/C mice, namely C.A-21 and A.C-20. C.A-21 mice are the counterpart of C.AL-20 mice. They are BALB/C mice with the A/J heavy chain locus (Ighe) instead of the AL/N heavy chain locus (Igho). A.C-20 congenic mice are A/J mice carrying the BALB/C heavy chain locus (Ighd). Anti-arsonate responses of these congenic mice have been compared with the anti-arsonate responses developed in C.AL-20 and (BALB/C × A/J) F1 hybrids.

From the results depicted in Table 1, it is clear that idiotype expression is governed mainly by the Igh locus. Anti-idiotypic monoclonal antibodies and anti-idiotypic polyclonal reagents lead to the same conclusions drawn previously.

Nevertheless, some intriguing reports have mentioned that BALB/C produced CRI positive molecules even after arsonate injection [60, 76, 77]. These observations are not easily reconciled since CRI positively is associated with presence of a strain specific VH gene segment.

Using the idiotypic cascade first studied in rabbits, we have shown all BALB/C mice can express high amounts of anti-arsonate antibodies which bear the CRIA serologic determinants [78]. Sera react strongly with E4, E3 and H8 anti-idiotypic monoclonal antibodies but are negative with the 2D3 monoclonal antibody [60]. Briefly, BALB/C mice manipulated with the idiotypic cascade were first immunized with rabbit anti-CRI rendered specific for idiotypic determinants by repeated passages over sepharose columns coupled with normal A/J globulins, followed by adsorption on a column of sepharose coupled to BALB/C anti-arsonate antibodies. Then anti-CRI treated BALB/C were injected with arsonate conjugated to KLH.

Two CRIA positive hybridoma products derived from BALB/C mice have been sequenced. These molecules utilize the same light chain structures as A/J CRIA positive antibodies (VK10.1 and JK1). Their D segments are remarkably homologous to the DFL16.1 gene segment of A/J CRIA positive antibodies, but their heavy chain VH gene segment is totally different from the VHIdCR11 and belongs to another VH gene family, namely VHGAM3.8. For this reason the BALB/C CRIA is termed CRIA-like [79, 80].

The logical extension of the BALB/C study was the generation of CRIA idiotype positive molecules in mice lacking both crucial alleles. The C.C58 congenic strain was chosen and idiotypically manipulated. C.C58 were able to produce CRIA-like antibodies serologically indistinguishable from BALB/C CRIA-like antibodies [81]. These data suggest an inappropriate light chain locus can supply a light chain to sustain the expression of CRIA-like positive molecules.

To determine the light chain sequence used by the C.C58 CRIA-like antibodies, a less restrictive approach was employed as the double congenic C.C58.AL-20 strain. C.C58.AL-20 mice are BALB/C mice carrying the AL/N heavy chains and the C58 light chains. Both in serum and hybridoma, CRIA-like molecules were easily detected after idiotypic manipulation. Structural analysis revealed the light chains recruited in the C.C58.AL-20 response were the closest counterparts of the A/J and BALB/C light chains present in C58 strain [82]. Studies in Capra's laboratory have shown the AKR (and C.C58) VK10.1 gene segment could not probably support the idiotype expression because the CDR region was very different from the A/J VK10.1 gene segment. The rest of the VK10.1 gene segment is virtually identical to the A/J VK10.1 gene segment [75]. Three of four hybridomas sequenced support this conclusion since the third hypervariable regions are markedly mutated (one actually mutated towards the A/J germline sequence). However, one hybridoma has a completely germline third hypervariable region. Another striking observation in these monoclonal antibodies was the use of both VH gene segments, the BALB/C VGAM3.8 and the canonical A/J VHIdCR11 to encode C.C58.AL-20 idiotype positive molecules.

Studies on idiotypically manipulated mice allow us to draw at least two major conclusions:

1 Molecules that share serologic specificities can have vastly different primary structures.
2 The immune system is extremely flexible and possesses a large capacity to generate antibodies to virtually any structure by using various combinations of available gene segments, junctional variations, and somatic mutations.

Table 1. Idiotypic Analyses of Anti-arsonate Responses in Congenic Strains

	ARS	2D3	E4	E3	7B7
A/J	11[a]	2900[b]	3200	1200	400
	12	2400	3300	1200	320
	9.5	1400	1000	450	400
	10	1100	100	200	250
	9	1500	1000	900	340
	6	700	1100	1000	1200
	3	180	c	40	–
	4	1300	720	700	10
	5	160	260	200	10
C.A-21	0.2	24	–	15	5
	5.4	1700	1640	2410	810
	2	130	50	60	50
	0.2	20	–	20	–
	0.5	800	310	540	250
	6.8	510	80	240	60
	5.6	520	500	820	280
	3	530	600	600	220
	6.5	460	–	90	4
C.AL-20	2.3	390	250	280	180
	1.4	360	120	90	160
	1.5	620	380	250	130
	2	70	–	20	40
	4.3	620	250	340	10
	1.1	360	290	260	30
	1.8	490	470	960	150
	0.2	–	–	30	–
	2	850	230	1300	340
	2.2	360	210	450	40
	1.9	60	20	10	20
	5.8	320	160	130	10
	4.4	1240	830	630	170
	1.7	320	140	100	70

	ARS	2D3	E4	E3	7B7
BALB/C	5.2	–	–	9	–
	4	–	–	–	–
	5.7	–	–	–	–
	8.8	–	40	–	–
	12	–	140	–	–
	10	–	–	–	–
	8.2	–	65	7	–
	1.7	–	–	–	–
	4	–	–	–	N.D.
	7.7	–	260	–	N.D.
A.C-20	14.9	–	–	–	–
	12	–	–	–	–
	14.1	–	–	–	–
	27	–	260	6	–
	22	–	230	20	–
	22	–	170	–	–
	25.6	–	–	20	–
	20	–	–	–	–
	18	–	170	15	–
	43	–	–	–	–
	38	–	1140	20	–
CAF1	3.3	630	130	300	34
	16.5	1260	510	105	34
	10.2	2240	560	450	–
	6.2	420	230	200	54
	10.6	–	–	–	–
	16	60	90	70	50
	10	170	–	–	8
	22.5	3780	4700	2810	80
	20	490	2900	470	54
	18.2	1100	940	870	20

Results are given for individual serum samples obtained on day 21 or 28 of the secondary anti-arsonate response.
[a] Concentrations of anti-arsonate antibody in mg/ml (3665 equivalent).
[b] Concentrations of CRIA idiotope (2D3, E4, E3, 7B7) in µg/ml (3665 equivalent).
[c] Level of idiotypic positive antibodies was under the detection limit of the assay. The limits were 2D3 7 µg/ml, E4 10 µg/ml, E3 3 µg/ml and 7B7 1 µg/ml.
N.D. – not done.

Nevertheless, these studies lead us to ask why some idiotypes remain private and others become recurrent. Most popular explanations are based on the clonal selection theory; others refer to the idiotypic network.

To understand the rules of the idiotypic selection, we have studied CRIA and CRIA-like idiotype expressions in a large panel of recombinant inbred strains between A/J and BALB/C immunized with Ars-KLH. R. Riblet had derived 12 recombinant inbred strains named AXC1 to AXC12. Recombinant inbred strains AXC1 to AXC6 have the upstream part of the BALB/C Igh locus while the downstream (the most D proximal) part is of A/J origin. The genetic content of AXC7 to AXC12 contains the upstream part of the A/J Igh locus and the BALB/C downstream part. AXC7 to AXC12 strains contain the VHIdCR11 of A/J, but the D gene segments come from BALB/C (BALB/C DFL16.1). Their anti-arsonate responses are dominated by the CRIA idiotype as the A/J anti-arsonate response. The 2D3 similar expression between AXC7 to AXC12 and A/J indicates that the VHIdCR11 is used.

We have shown previously that the private CRIA-like idiotype of BALB/C becomes recurrent in the recombinant inbred strain AXC1 that possesses part of the VH from BALB/C and the D gene segments from A/J [83]. Thus, a private idiotype can become recurrent after genetic shuffling. However, the AXC1 CRIA-like idiotype is not dominant as the A/J CRIA idiotype. At least 80% of A/J mice express the CRIA idiotype in anti-arsonate response. Only 1 or 2% of BALB/C mice make significant amounts of CRIA-like idiotype after antigen immunization, while in the AXC1 mice more than 30% of the mice synthesize clearly the CRIA-like idiotype. Another 30% produce low but significant amounts of the CRIA-like idiotype. The last third is negative for CRIA-like expression. The other recombinant inbred strains (AXC2–AXC6) with the AXC1 genetic design develop an anti-arsonate response similar to the one described in AXC1.

To reveal putative regulatory mechanisms that influence the expression of the CRIA-like idiotype, (AXC1 × BALB/C) F1 hybrid mice have been immunized with arsonate. Unexpectedly, we observed a complete inhibition of the CRIA-like idiotype expression suggesting a priori two explanations:

1   Clonal competition: BALB/C mice make another dominant idiotype, the CRIC. It is therefore possible that if the CRIC idiotype has a better affinity for arsonate than CRIA-like, the CRIC clones will compete better for the antigen and the CRIA-like clones will no more be stimulated with antigen.
2   Other genes outside the Igh or Igl loci could influence the fate of idiotype expression.

We have measured both CRIA-like and CRIC idiotype expressions in (AXC1 × BALB/C) F1 and homozygous mice. Data showed an equal level of CRIC idiotype expression in (AXC1 × BALB/C) F1, CRIA-like positive AXC1, CRIA-like negative AXC1, and BALB/C. The disappearance of CRIA-like idiotype in (AXC1 × BALB/C) F1 was not due to the dominance of CRIC. The first explanation is clearly not valid.

To understand this phenomenon further, we performed backcross experiments between (AXC1 × BALB/C) F1 and AXC1. AXC1 and BALB/C mice have a polymorphism at IgG2a isotype that allowed the backcrossed mice to be typed for their IgCH locus. Thirty-four of 39 heterozygote mice were negative for idiotype expression. In 73 homozygote mice, 38% were found positive for idiotype, a percentage very close to those observed in AXC1 mice (Table 2).

These data can be explained simply by stating that the Igh locus dictates idiotype expression. From congenic strains and recombinant inbred strains, we could not detect a profound influence of background genes. The Igh locus dominates the rules of idiotype expression.

A major question that remains is "What is the reason for CRIA-like extinction in F1 mice?" One possible explanation is based on the fact that DFL16.1 gene segments of the strains differ by one amino acid replacement. The DFL16.1 from A/J mice contains glycine (position 104) while the D segment from BALB/C has a serine at the same position. The AXC1 strain has the D gene segment from A/J; the AXC7 to AXC12 strains have the D from BALB/C. It seems, therefore, that the results can be explained if we suppose that the substitution glycine-serine has dramatic consequences on the affinity for arsonate or that an idiotope could be localized in that area between glycine and serine.

A detailed analysis based on the three-dimensional structure of the CRIA and the predictive properties of a computer graphics program has been done (Hasemann, personal communication): this analysis predicts that this replacement should be neutral and should not affect the affinity of the antibody binding site. However, a site-directed mutagenesis analysis is needed to settle the matter. At this stage the bulk of data suggests that idiotype expression is governed by genetic polymorphism. It is nevertheless surprising that the F1 data cannot be explained by the dominance of the CRIC idiotype.

Regulatory Influences in the Arsonate System

It is frequently assumed that idiotype dominance can be explained by a minimal model involving antigen alone. The usual model posits that all B-lymphocytes participating in the response compete with one another for a limited supply of antigen, with survival or preferential expansion of high affinity clones. Although it is beyond doubt that antigenic selection plays an important role, much data indicate the rules of the game are more complex. For example, the introduction of somatically mutated V region with an unusually high affinity for arsonate in the pre-immune repertoire for A/J mice did not affect many aspects of antigen driven B-cell differentiation in the endogenous V gene expressing clones, although the unmutated antibody repertoire is of 100-fold lower affinity. No dominance of these high affinity clones was observed in the primary and secondary repertoires [84]. This, of course, suggests affinity alone cannot dictate dominance.

Our data suggest that idiotype dominance, occurring in nearly 90% of A/J mice immunized with Ars-KLH, can be broken surprisingly easily by various means while the level of anti-arsonate antibodies is not affected. For example, the treatment at birth of A/J mice with anti-μ antibodies leads to the disappearance of idiotype dominance when these mice are subsequently injected with Ars-KLH after the recovery of a normal FACS profile for B-lymphocytes. In these animals the level of anti-arsonate antibodies is normal. Similar results are obtained when

Table 2. CRIA-like Idiotype Expression in AXC1, (AXC1 BALB/C) F1 and (F1 × AXC1) F2 Mice

Strain	AXC1	BALB/C	(AXC1×BALB/c)F1	(F1 × AXC1)F2	
IghC	e/e	a/a	a/e	a/e	e/e
N° of mice	85	30	29	39	73
CRIA-like ++[a]	28[d] E3 (2–100)[e] E4 (2–103)	1 E3(73) E4 (19)	0	1 E3 (55) E4 (15)	28 E3 (4–105) E4 (20–160)
CRIA-like +/−[b]	23 E3 (112–500) E4 (100–535)	3 E3 (1.4×10^3–15×10^3) E4 (1.2×10^3–9.4×10^3)	6 E3 (150–260) E4 (90–630)	4 E3 (44–215) E4 (100–265)	21 E3 (130–400) E4(145–1.8×10^3)
CRIA-like −[c]	34	26	23	34	24

Mice were tested on the secondary response day 28.
[a] ++ mice have more than 5% of CRIA-like anti-arsonate Ab;
[b] +/− mice have less than 5% of CRIA-like anti-arsonate Ab;
[c] − mice have less than 1% of CRIA-like anti-arsonate Ab;
[d] Number of mice;
[e] Values inside brackets represent range of weight (ng) anti-arsonate Ab to obtain 50% inhibition on Ab2m assays.

antigen is present at birth. In this case, antigen (Ars-dHGG) is given to mothers during the first day following delivery [85].

Another experimental strategy leading to CRIA disappearance involves the transfer of naïve B-lymphocytes in syngeneic irradiated recipients or in irradiated recipients with hind limbs partially shielded to allow auto reconstitution [86–89].

Detailed molecular and histological studies have been made on these animals. While the level of anti-arsonate antibodies upon a secondary immunization is normal, there is no selection of the memory idiotype. The maturation of affinity and the frequency of somatic mutations are reduced. Isotype switching and the development of full-blown germinal centers are delayed. Some components of immunological memory are present (rise in antibody level and the kinetics of antibody response) while some other memory properties are lost or impaired (selection of the memory idiotype, affinity maturation, development of germinal center).

Another striking phenomenon is the opposite behavior of different idiotypes after treatment of adult A/J mice with anti-μ or anti-δ antibodies. In addition to CRIA, the memory idiotype, these studies concern another idiotype of the arsonate system, the CRIC idiotype, which is present throughout the response with no preferential temporal pattern [43].

Adult A/J mice were injected several times with anti-μ or anti-δ antibodies. These mice were subsequently immunized with antigen several times, the first injection of antigen given under the antibody treatment.

Injections of anti-μ antibodies led to a striking enhancement of the memory idiotype in the primary response and the usual dominance of CRIA in the secondary response. By contrast, the treatment with anti-δ leads to a dramatic decrease of the CRIA idiotype while the CRIC idiotype is unaffected. Strikingly, the injections of anti-μ or anti-δ lead to a strong modification in the B-lymphocyte subsets: more precisely, anti-μ treatment promotes a striking enhancement of the HSA^{low} subset while anti-δ treatment enhances significantly the HSA^{high} compartment.

Interestingly, Klinman and his colleagues have shown naïve B2 lymphocytes can be subdivided into different subsets, including the HSA^{high} subset mainly involved in primary responses and the HSA^{low} subset containing the precursors of some memory cells [89, 90]. A semi-quantitative PCR analysis performed on the B-lymphocyte subsets in naïve A/J mice reveals that the presence of CRIA transcripts is mainly associated with the HSA^{low} compartment while CRIC transcripts are mainly associated with HSA^{high} subset. Altogether these data leave open the possibility that secondary B-cell lineage is selected in the preimmune repertoire by internal images within the idiotype network. These data also suggest that the immune system is endowed with several kinds of memory, one stemming from the clonal expansion and differentiation of the primary B-cell subset (HSA^{high}), the second developing from the secondary B-cell subset (HSA^{low}).

The first kind of memory is the one predominating in autoreconstituted irradiated mice. In these irradiated animals the level of anti-arsonate antibodies upon a secondary immunization is normal, but there is no selection of the CRIA memory idiotype. Some components of immunological memory are present (the rise and kinetics of antibody concentration) while other memory properties are lost or impaired (development of germinal centers, selection of the memory idiotype, affinity maturation). These lost properties can be attributed to the HSA^{low} subset (secondary B-cell lineage).

Studies performed by Klinman's group have associated the HSA^{low} subset with somatic mutations [91]. Our data fit well with those of Klinman group [89, 90].

Some data already suggest positive selection during the development of B-lymphocytes.

Gu *et al.* [92] have shown the expression of unmutated genes belonging to the J558 V_H family is remarkably different when adults are compared to neonates. Lam *et al.* [93] have convincingly demonstrated that the survival of naïve B-lymphocytes depends on the presence of BCR. Furthermore, the V region of BCR is essential for B-cell survival [3].

Several mechanisms, not necessarily exclusive, could account for these findings [94].

First, constitutive signalling without the need for an external ligand can be considered. The BCR *per se* would deliver maintenance signals necessary for B-cell survival. This proposal has been favored in papers suggesting that the selection within the B1 subset depends on the density of surface immunoglobulin [95].

However, recent data indicate that the presence of the BCR is not just merely sufficient. The BCR specificity determines the geographical location and the subset of B-lymphocytes. Therefore, ligand recognition seems necessary for B-cell preferential survival and maintenance. B-lymphocytes like T-lymphocytes are submitted to a process of positive selection. These ligands could be external (i.e., bacteria) or internal (self-antigens or idiotypic partners).

In at least one case, positive selection of B-cells into the B1 subset depends critically on the presence of a self-antigen (Thy1.2) since the analysis of mice, in which the gene coding for the self-antigen was inactivated, shows no preferential selection into the B1 subset [96]. Recent data suggest that the marginal zone B-cell repertoire is positively selected [97].

At this stage, for the arsonate system, we conclude that the CRI$_A$ repertoire is positively selected into a B2 subset, the HSA^{low} subset. Can this selection be explained by idiotypic cascades operating in ontogeny or, in other words, by idiotypic networks?

We have tried to evaluate this hypothesis using the following scheme. Since idiotypic networks depend critically on Ab1-Ab2 interactions, we asked what would happen to the immune system of A/J mice if we delete or inactivate auto-anti-idiotypic B-lymphocytes in the pre-immune repertoire.

Therefore, we tried to inactivate such B-lymphocytes by injecting newborn A/J mice with deleting antibodies specific for shared idiotopes of anti Ab2 antibodies (in fact, rabbit polyclonal Ab3 antibodies raised against murine Ab2) or with pre-immune sera from the same rabbits [37]. At the age of 2 months, these A/J mice were immunized with the Ars-KLH conjugate. The level of anti-arsonate antibodies was normal but the idiotype dominance was lost. It can be objected that the rabbit Ab2 antibodies have perhaps primed auto Ab2 lymphocytes instead of deleting them. However, A/J mice never develop antibodies against rabbit immunoglobulins and no precursors of autoantiidiotypic B-lymphocytes could be detected.

We conclude that auto Ab2 lymphocyte presence at birth is essential for CRIA dominance in the adult.

Other findings support the hypothesis of positive selection of some B-lympho-cytes by idiotypic networks [6, 98]. An IgH chain transgene was placed into the germ line of mice homozygous for deletion in the necessary JH gene segments. The light chains expressed were sequenced from both immature and mature B-cell subpopulations. There was a selection for particular light chain sequences and the set of light chains was dependent on the heavy chain transgene chosen. The same phenomenon was observed in gnotobiotic mice and a role for terminal deoxynu-cleotidyl transferase (TdT) was excluded. Thus it was proposed that "Jerne idio-typic network . . . actually can act on the naïve B-cell repertoire to positively select certain heavy, light chain pairs over others." Interestingly, this positive selection is not observed in mice where the genetically engineered heavy chain cannot be secreted, implying that positive selection is at least partly due to soluble antibody [99]. Likewise, using an "oligoclonal" model, it was shown that the mice trans-genic for given μ chain (H3) and deficient for K chain expression display a mature B-cell repertoire largely dominated by the H3/λ1 pair, despite the fact that the four λ chains are present in the immature B-cell compartment. Further experi-ments using the SLJ λ1 deficiency led the authors to conclude that the H3/λ1 dominance is due to positive selection and not to a negative selection of other H3/λ chain combination [98]. Most splenic B-cells in mice that lack Aiolos are mature IgD^{high} IgM^{low} follicular B-lymphocytes. Probably maturation signals delivered through the BCR are enhanced when the zinc transcription factor Aiolos is absent. This enhanced maturation of follicular B-cells is accompanied by the absence of marginal zone B-cells. In the words of the authors [100], these data sup-port the notion that antigen (in contrast to "tonic" signals) drive the development of naïve B-cells. Splenic marginal zone B-cells join B1 B-cells to generate a massive wave of IgM producing plamablasts in the first phase of a primary response toward particular bacterial antigen. It has been proposed that marginal zone B-cells and B1 cells represent a "natural memory" bridging the early innate and the later adaptive immune response [101].

V. IMMUNOLOGICAL CONSCIOUSNESS

The complexities and properties of the immune and nervous systems have often been compared. Both systems rest upon a huge number of cells; both are predetermined to predict the imprevisible and both display memory, which represent the adaptation to the internal and external environments. A further analogy can be found in the recent discovery of protocadherins (PCAD). PCAD are made up of V and C exons and contain three classes. In the α class, 15 Vα parts, in the β class 15 functional Vβ parts and in the γ class 22 functional Vγ parts can be linked to the corresponding C parts. If one assumes homophilic binding, a three-dimensional structure made up of 4950 neurons ($15 \times 15 \times 22$) emerges from one stem cell (for a recent review see [102]).

Recently, problems associated with understanding consciousness in the brain have been the subject of several papers and books [103–107].

Some structures in the brain deal with emotions and feelings. Other structures have evolved allowing Cartesian decisions (the Boolean brain). In the somatic self-marker hypothesis, Antonio Damasio – on the basis of experimental findings on patients – proposes the absence of emotions can lead to a severe impairment in the ability of rationale decision-making. Emotions are biologically indispensable for logical deductions. High reason depends on low brain (so to speak). In the same vein, Suzanne Greenfield [108] writes: *"Computers cannot think because computers do not have emotions"* (2000).

Much like the three stages in the evolution of the brain, we can distinguish three stages in the evolution of immunity.

Early in evolution, the so-called innate immune system appeared (devoid of the diversity of immunological receptors – immunoglobulins and T-cell receptors) using pattern recognition receptors which recognize molecular signatures of pathogens or stressed self-molecules (heat shock proteins...) [6, 109]. Ligand recognition by theses receptors allows the activation of macrophages and other cells which will destroy the pathogen or the damaged self-molecules.

A second immune system was built by the introduction of a bacterial transposase gene allowing the generation of a large array of V regions. Like in the multigene family of odorant receptors, expression of specific receptors became highly restricted inside one cell. This second immune system is not independent of the first but functions only in an efficient way if the first immune system has been alerted. This has been achieved by linking the transduction pathways of the pattern recognition receptors to those of the first (antigen receptor) and second signals (costimulatory signals: B7 family, CD40, OX40...). Only cells alerted by danger signals will display a sufficient amount of costimulatory signals necessary to activate lymphocytes recognized on antigen.

Just as the Cartesian brain cannot properly function if the emotional brain has been damaged, the immune system cannot mount an adequate specific immune response if danger signals are absent. Danger signals furnish feelings to the immune system.

As soon as diversity exploded, the immune system had to cope with the inherent noisy background of network interaction (see above). Then came the third immune system playing with the combinations of the past (the self+maternal immunoglobulins) to predict the future, thereby building an anti-antiself pre-memory compartment.

Like Anatonio Damasio, we have called this "memories of the future" and propose these memories of the future reside at least partially in the HSA^{low} B-cell subset.

The idiotype network in this context will have two functions: building a pre-memory B-cell subset to allow maternal imprinting and helping in maintaining the diversity of germ line genes.

Let us end this chapter with a quotation from Antonio Damasio's remarkable book, *Descartes Error* (1994).

> In some species, nonhuman and even nonprimate, in which memory, reasoning and creativity are limited, there are nonetheless manifestations of complex social behavior whose neural control must be innate. Insects – ants and bees in particular – offer dramatic examples of social cooperation that might easily put to shame the United Nations General Assembly most any day. Close to home, mammals abound in such manifestations, and the behaviors of wolves, dolphins and vampire bats, among other species, even suggest an ethical structure. It is apparent that humans possess some of those same innate

mechanisms and that such mechanisms are the likely basis for some ethical structures used by humans. The most elaborate social conventions and ethical structures by which we live, however, must have arisen culturally and been transmitted likewise.

If that is the case, one may wonder: what was the trigger for the cultural development of such strategies? It is likely they evolved as a means to cope with suffering experienced by individuals whose capacity to remember the past and anticipate the future had attained a remarkable development. In other words, the strategies evolved in individuals able to realize that their survival was threatened or that the quality of their post-survival life could be bettered. Such strategies could have evolved only in the few species whose brains were structured to permit the following. First, a large capacity to memorize categories of objects and events, and to memorize unique objects and events, that is, to establish dispositional representations of entities and events at the level of categories and at unique levels. Second, a large capacity for manipulating the components of those memorized representations and fashioning new creations by means of novel combinations. The most immediately useful variety of those creations consisted of imagined scenarios, the anticipation of outcomes of actions, the formulation of future plans, and the design of new goals that can enhance survival. Third, a large capacity to memorize the new creations described above, that is, the anticipated outcomes, the new plans and the new goals. I call those memorized creation "memories of the future."

If enhanced knowledge of the experience past and the anticipated future was the reason social strategies had to be created to cope with suffering, we still must explain why suffering arose in the first place. And for that we must consider the biologically prescribed sense of pain as well as its opposite – pleasure. The curious thing is, of course, that the biological mechanisms behind what we now call pain and pleasure were also an important reason the innate instruments of survival were selected and simply mean that the same simple device, applied to systems with very different orders of complexity and in different circumstances, leads to different but related results. The immune system, the hypothalamus, the ventromedial frontal cortices, and the Bill of Rights have the same root cause.

ACKNOWLEDGMENTS

This work was supported by the Pole d'Attraction Interuniversitaires from the Belgian Government. The authors wish to thank Prof. D. Capra and M. Zanetti for their precious help and suggestions.

REFERENCES

1. Coutinho, A., Salaun, J., Corbel, C., Bandeira, A., and Le Douarin, N. (1993). The role of thymic epithelium in the establishment of transplantation tolerance. *Immunol Rev.* **133**, 225–40.
2. Shevach, E.M. (2001). Certified professionals: CD4(+)CD25(+) suppressor T cells. *J. Exp. Med.* **193**, F41–6.

3. Rosado, M.M., and Freitas, A.A. (1998). The role of the B cell receptor V region in peripheral B cell survival. *Eur. J. Immunol.* **28**, 2685–93.

4. Marshall, E. (1996). Disputed results now just a footnote. *Science* **273**, 174–5.

5. Cohn, M. (1994). The wisdom of insight. *Ann. Rev. Immunol.* **12**, 1–62.

6. Janeway, C.A., Jr. (2001). Inaugural Article: How the immune system works to protect the host from infection: A personal view. *Proc. Natl. Acad. Sci. USA.* **98**, 7461–8.

7. Holmberg, D., Portnoi, D., Jacquemart, F., Forsgren, S., Araujo, P., Andrade, L., Lundqvist, I., and Coutinho, A. (1986). The repertoire of naturally activated B-cells suggests the functionality of the idiotypic network. *Ann. Inst. Pasteur Immunol.* **137C**, 85–7.

8. Slaoui, M., Urbain-Vansanten, G., Demeur, C., Leo, O., Marvel, J., Moser, M., Tassignon, J., Greene, M.I., Urbain, J. (1986). Idiotypic games within the immune network. *Immunol. Rev.* **90**, 73–91.

9. Urbain, J., Brait, M., De Wit, D., Ismaili, J., Leo, O., Ryelandt, M., Tassignon, J., Vansanten-Urbain, G., Van Acker, A., Willems, F. (1992). B cell subsets, idiotype selection: positive selection for some B lymphocytes? *Int. Rev. Immunol.* **8**, 259–67.

10. Coutinho, A., Freitas, A.A., Holmberg, D., and Grandien, A. (1992). Expression and selection of murine antibody repertoires. *Int. Rev. Immunol.* **8**, 173–87.

11. Cohn, M. (1986). The concept of functional idiotype network mocks all and comforts none. *Am. Immunol.* **137C**, 64–76.

12. Lemke, H., and Lange, H. (1999). Is there a maternally induced immunological imprinting phase a la Konrad Lorenz? *Scand. J. Immunol.* **50**, 348–54.

13. Steele, E.J., Lindley, R., and Blanden, R. (1998). Lamarck's signature. Reading, Massachusetts, *Frontier of Science*.

14. Urbain, J., Wuilmart, C., and Cazenave, P.A., (1981). Idiotypic regulation in immune networks. *Contemp. Top. Mol. Immunol.* **8**, 113–48.

15. Urbain, J., Brait, M., Bruyns, C., Demeur, C., Dubois, P., Francotte, M., Franssen, J.D., Hiernaux, J., Leo, O., and Marvel, J. (1985). The idiotypic network: order from the beginning or order out of chaos? *Curr. Top. Microbiol. Immunol.* **119**, 127–42.

16. Kearney, J.F., Bartels, J., Hamilton, A.M., Lehuen, A., Solvason, N., and Vakil, M. (1992). Development and function of the early B cell repertoire. *Int. Rev. Immunol.* **8**, 247–57.

17. Lemke, H., and Lange, H. (2001). *Two basic functions of the idiotypic network*.

18. Agrawal, A., Laforsch, C., and Tollrian R. (1999). Transgenerational induction of defences in animals and plants. *Nature* **401**, 60–63.

19. Zinkernagel, R.M. (2000). *Immunol. Today* **21**, 422–3.

20. Cazenave, P.A. (1977). Idiotypic-anti-idiotypic regulation of antibody synthesis in rabbits. *Proc. Natl. Acad. Sci. USA* **74**, 512–15.

21. Urbain, J., Wikler, M., Franssen, J.D., and Collignon, C. (1977). Idiotypic regulation of the immune system by the induction of antibodies against anti-idiotypic antibodies. *Proc. Natl. Acad. Sci. USA.* **74**, 5126–30.

22. Urbain, J., Francotte, M., Franssen, J.D., Hiernaux, J., Leo, O., Moser, M., Slaoui, M., Urbain-Vansanten, G., Van Acker, A., and Wikler, M. (1983). From clonal selection to immune networks: induction of silent idiotypes. *Ann. NY Acad. Sci.* **418**, 1–8.

23. Wikler, M., Franssen, J.D., Collignon, C., Leo, O., Mariame, B., Van de Walle, P., De Groote, D., and Urbain, J. (1979). Idiotypic regulation of the immune system. Common idiotypic specificities between idiotypes and antibodies raised against anti-idiotypic antibodies in rabbits. *J. Exp. Med.* **150**, 184–95.

24. Sege, K., and Peterson, P.A. (1978). Anti-idiotypic antibodies against anti-vitamin A transporting protein react with prealbumin. *Nature* **271**, 167–8.

25. Jerne, N.K., Roland, J., and Cazenave, P.A. (1982). Recurrent idiotopes and internal images. *EMBO. J.* **1**, 243–7.

26. Urbain, J., Slaoui, M., and Leo, O. (1982). Idiotypes, recurrent idiotypes and internal images. *Ann. Immunol.* (Paris). **133D**, 179–89.

27. Francotte, M., and Urbain, J. (1985). Enhancement of antibody response by mouse dendritic cells pulsed with tobacco mosaic virus or with rabbit anti-idiotypic antibodies raised against a private rabbit idiotype. *Proc. Natl. Acad. Sci.* USA. **82**, 8149–52.

28. Fougereau, M., and Schiff, C. (1988). Breaking the first circle. *Immunol. Rev.* **105**, 69–84.

29. Goldbaum, F., Velisovsky, C., Dall'acqua, N., Fossatica, Fields, B.A., Braden, B.C., Poljak, R., and Mariuzza, R. (1997). Three-dimensional structure of an idiotype-anti-idiotope complex. *Proc. Natl Acad. Sci.* **94**, 8697–8701.

30. Ban, N., Escobar, C., Hasel, K., Day, J., Greenwood, A., and McPherson, A. (1995). Structure of an anti-idiotype Fab against feline peritonitis virus neutralizing antibody and a comparison with the complexed Fab. *FASEB J.* 107–114.

31. Friboulet, A., Izadyar, L., Avalle, B., Roseto, A., and Thomas, D. (1995). Anti-idiotypic antibodies as functional internal images of enzyme-active sites. *Ann. NY. Acad. Sci.* **750**, 265–70.

32. Rodkey, L.S. (1974). Studies of idiotypic antibodies. Production and characterization of autoantiidiotypic antisera. *J. Exp. Med.* **139**, 712–20.

33. Wuilmart, C., Wikler, M., and Urbain, J. (1979). Induction of autoanti-idiotypic antibodies and effects on the subsequent immune response. *Mol. Immunol.* **16**, 1085–92.

34. Kluskens, L., and Kohler, H. (1974). Regulation of immune response by autogenous antibody against receptor. *Proc. Natl. Acad. Sci.* USA. **71**, 5083–7.

35. Tasiaux, N., Leuwenkroon, R., Bruyns, C., and Urbain, J. (1978). Possible occurrence and meaning of lymphocytes bearing autoanti-idiotypic receptors during the immune response. *Eur. J. Immunol.* **8**, 464–8.

36. Lange, H., and Lemke, H. (1996). Induction of a non-oscillating, long-lasting humoral immune response to an internal network antigen. *Int. Immunol.* **8**, 683–8.

37. Ismaili, J., Brait, M., Leo, O., and Urbain, J. (1995). Assessment of a functional role of auto-anti-idiotypes in idiotype dominance. *Eur. J. Immunol.* **25**, 830–7.

38. Silverstein, A. (1989). *A history of immunology.* Acad Press.

39. Gell, P.G., and Kelus, A.S. (1967). Anti-antibodies. *Adv. Immunol.* **6**, 461–78.

40. Jerne, N.K. (1973). The immune system. *Sci. Am.* **229**, 52–60.

41. Jerne, N.K. (1974). Towards a network theory of the immune system. *Ann. Immunol.* (Paris). **125C**, 373–89.

42. Urbain, J. (1976). Idiotypes, expression of antibody diversity and network concepts. *Ann. Immunol.* (Paris). **127**, 357–74.

43. Masungi Luko C., Vansanten, G., Ryelandt, M., Denis, O., Wuilmart, C., Andris, F., Van Acker, A., Brait, M., Cloquet, J.P., Ismaili, N., Nisol, F., Latinne, D., Brown, A., Leo, O., Bazin, H., and Urbain, J. (2000). Distinct VH repertoires in primary and secondary B cell lymphocyte subsets in the preimmune repertoire of A/J mice: the CRI-A idiotype is preferentially associated with the HSA(low) B cell subset. *Eur. J. Immunol.* **30**, 2312–22.

44. Jordan, M.S., Riley, M.P., von Boehmer, H., and Caton, A.J. (2000). Anergy and suppression regulate CD4(+) T cell responses to a self peptide. *Eur. J. Immunol.* **30**, 136–44.

45. Van Acker, A., Urbain-Vansanten, G., De Vos-Cloetens, C., Tasiaux, N., and Urbain, J. (1979). Synthesis of high affinity antibodies in irradiated rabbits grafted with allogeneic cells from hyperimmune donors. *Ann. Immunol.* (Paris). **130C**, 385–96.

46. Wikler, M., Demeur, C., Dewasme, G., and Urbain, J. (1980). Immunoregulatory role of maternal idiotypes. Ontogeny of immune networks. *J. Exp. Med.* **152**, 1024–35.

47. Montesano, M.A., Colley, D.G., Eloi-Santos, S., Freeman, G.L. Jr., and Secor, W.E. (1999). Neonatal idiotypic exposure alters subsequent cytokine, pathology, and survival patterns in experimental Schistosoma mansoni infections. *J. Exp. Med.* **189**, 637–45.

48. Lange, H., Kobarg, J., Yazynin, S., Solterbeck, M., Henningsen, M., Hansen, H., and Lemke, H. (1999). Genetic analysis of the maternally induced affinity enhancement in the non-Ox1 idiotypic antibody repertoire of the primary immune response to 2-phenyloxazolone. *Scand. J. Immunol.* **49**, 55–66.

49. Forni, L., Coutinho, A., Kohler, G., and Jerne, N.K. (1980). IgM antibodies induce the production of antibodies of the same specificity. *Proc. Natl. Acad. Sci. USA* **77**, 1125–8.
50. Martinez, C., Toribio, M.L., De la Hera, A., Cazenave, P.A., and Coutinho, A. (1986). Maternal transmission of idiotypic network interactions selecting available T cell repertoires. *Eur. J. Immunol.* **16**, 1445–7.
51. Kuettner, M.G., Wang, A.L., and Nisonoff, A. (1972). Quantitative investigations of idiotypic antibodies. VI. Idiotypic specificity as a potential genetic marker for the variable regions of mouse immunoglobulin polypeptide chains. *J. Exp. Med.* **135**, 579–95.
52. Rathbun, G., Sanz, I., Meek, K., Tucker, P., and Capra, J.D. (1988). The molecular genetics of the arsonate idiotypic system of A/J mice. *Adv. Immunol.* **42**, 95–164.
53. Robbins, P.F., Rosen, E.M., Haba, S., and Nisonoff, A. (1986). Relationship of VH and VL genes encoding three idiotypic families of anti-p-azobenzenearsonate antibodies. *Proc. Natl. Acad. Sci. USA* **83**, 1050–4.
54. Sharon, J., Gefter, M.L., Manser, T., Ptashne, M. (1986). Site-directed mutagenesis of an invariant amino acid residue at the variable-diversity segments junction of an antibody. *Proc. Natl. Acad. Sci. USA* **83**, 2628–31.
55. Sanz, I., and Capra, J.D. (1987). V kappa and J kappa gene segments of A/J Ars-A antibodies: somatic recombination generates the essential arginine at the junction of the variable and joining regions. *Proc. Natl. Acad. Sci. USA* **84**, 1085–9.
56. Manser, T., Wysocki, L.J., Margolies, M.N., and Gefter, M.L. (1987). Evolution of antibody variable region structure during the immune response. *Immunol. Rev.* **96**, 141–62.
57. Sharon, J., Gefter, M.L., Wysocki, L.J., and Margolies, M.N. (1989). Recurrent somatic mutations in mouse antibodies to p-azophenylarsonate increase affinity for hapten. *J. Immunol.* **142**, 596–601.
58. Parhami-Seren, B., Sharon, J., and Margolies, M.N. (1990). Structural characterization of H chain-associated idiotopes of anti-p-azophenylarsonate monoclonal antibodies. *J. Immunol.* **144**, 4426–33.
59. Wysocki, L.J., Liu, A.H., and Jena, P.K. (1998). Somatic mutagenesis and evolution of memory B-cells. *Curr. Top. Microbiol. Immunol.* **229**, 105–31.
60. Leo, O., Slaoui, M., Marvel, J., Milner, E.C., Hiernaux, J., Moser, M., Capra, J.D., Urbain, J. (1985). Idiotypic analysis of polyclonal and monoclonal anti-p-azophenylarsonate antibodies of BALB/c mice expressing the major cross-reactive idiotype of the A/J train. *J. Immunol.* **134**, 1734–9.
61. Jeske, D., Milner, E.C., Leo, O., Moser, M., Marvel, J., Urbain, J., and Capra, J.D. (1986). Molecular mapping of idiotopes of anti-arsonate antibodies. *J. Immunol.* **136**, 2568–74.
62. Hasemann, C.A., and Capra, J.D. (1991). Mutational analysis of the cross-reactive idiotype of the A strain mouse. *J. Immunol.* **147**, 3170–9.
63. Pawlak, L.L., Wang, A.L., and Nisonoff, A. (1973). Concentration of cross-reacting idiotypic specificities in unrelated mouse immunoglobulins. *J. Immunol.* **110**, 587–9.
64. Laskin, J.A., Gray, A., Nisonoff, A., Klinman, N.R., and Gottlieb, P.D. (1977). Segregation at a locus determining an immunoglobulin genetic marker for the light chain variable region affects inheritance of expression of an idiotype. *Proc. Natl. Acad. Sci. USA* **74**, 4600–4.
65. Brown, A.R., Estess, P., Lamoyi, E., Gill-Pazaris, L., Gottlieb, P.D., Capra, J.D., and Nisonoff, A. (1980). Studies of genetic control and microheterogeneity of an idiotype associated with anti-p-azophenylarsonate antibodies of A/J mice. *Prog. Clin. Biol. Res.* **42**, 231–47.
66. Edelman, G.M., and Gottlieb, P.D. (1970). A genetic marker in the variable region of light chains of mouse immunoglobulins. *Proc. Natl. Acad. Sci. USA* **67**, 1192–9.
67. Gottlieb, P.D. (1974). Genetic Correlation of a mouse light chain variable region marker with a thymocyte surface antigen. *J. Exp. Med.* **140**, 1432–7.
68. Gibson, D. (1976). Genetic polymorphism of mouse immunoglobulin light chains revealed by isoelectric focusing. *J. Exp. Med.* **144**, 298–303.
69. Goldrick, M.M., Boyd, R.T., Ponath, P.D., Lou, S.Y., and Gottlieb, P.D. (1985). Molecular genetic analysis of the V kappa Ser group associated with two mouse light

chain genetic markers. Complementary DNA cloning and southern hybridization analysis. *J. Exp. Med.* **162**, 713–28.

70. Boyd, R.T., Goldrick, M.M., and Gottlieb, P.D. (1986). Structural differences in a single gene encoding the V kappa Ser group of light chains explain the existence of two mouse light-chain genetic markers. *Proc. Natl. Acad. Sci. USA* **83**, 9134–8.

71. D'Hoostelaere, L., Huppi, K., Mock, B., Mallett, C., Gibson, D., Hilgers, J., and Potter, M. (1988). The organization of the immunoglobulin kappa locus in mice. *Curr. Top. Microbiol. Immunol.* **137**, 116–29.

72. Siekevitz. M., Gefter, M.L., Brodeur, P., Riblet, R., Marshak-Rothstein, A. (1982). The genetic basis of antibody production: the dominant anti-arsonate idiotype response of the strain A mouse. *Eur. J. Immunol.* **12**, 1023–32.

73. Siekevitz, M., Huang, S.Y., Gefter, M.L. (1983). The genetic basis of antibody production: a single heavy chain variable region gene encodes all molecules bearing the dominant anti-arsonate idiotype in the strain A mouse. *Eur. J. Immunol.* **13**, 123–32.

74. Meek, K., Hasemann, C., Pollok, B., Alkan, S.S., Brait, M., Slaoui, M., Urbain, J., and Capra, J.D. (1989). Structural characterization of antiidiotypic antibodies. Evidence that Ab2s are derived from the germline differently than Ab1s. *J. Exp. Med.* **169**, 519–33.

75. Kim, S.O., Sanz, I., Williams, C., Capra, J.D., and Gottlieb, P.D. (1991). Polymorphism in V kappa 10 genes encoding L chains of antibodies bearing the Ars-A and A48 cross-reactive idiotypes. *Immunogenetics* **34**, 231–41.

76. Sigal, N.H. (1982). Regulation of azophenylarsonate-specific repertoire expression. 1. Frequency of cross-reactive idiotype-positive B-cells in A/J and BALB/c mice. *J. Exp. Med.* **156**, 1352–65.

77. Lucas, A., and Henry, C. (1982). Expression of the major cross-reactive idiotype in a primary anti-azobenzenearsonate response. *J. Immunol.* **128**, 802–6.

78. Moser, M., Leo, O., Hiernaux, J., and Urbain, J. (1983). Idiotypic manipulation in mice: BALB/c mice can express the crossreactive idiotype of A/J mice. *Proc. Natl. Acad. Sci. USA* **80**, 4474–8.

79. Meek, K., Jeske, D., Slaoui, M., Leo, O., Urbain, J., and Capra, J.D. (1984a). Complete amino acid sequence of heavy chain variable regions derived from two monoclonal anti-p-azophenylarsonate antibodies of BALB/c mice expressing the major cross-reactive idiotype of the A/J strain. *J. Exp. Med.* **160**, 1070–86.

80. Meek, K., Sanz, I., Rathbun, G., Nisonoff, A., and Capra, J.D. (1984b) Identity of the V kappa 10-Ars-A gene segments of the A/J and BALB/c strains. *Proc. Natl. Acad. Sci. USA* **84**, 6244–8.

81. Marvel, J., Tassignon, J., Brait, M., Meek, K., Milner, E.C., Moser, M., Capra, J.D., and Urbain, J. (1987). The influence of V kappa gene polymorphism on the induction of silent idiotypes in the arsonate system. *Mol. Immunol.* **24**, 463–9.

82. Tassignon, J., Brait, M., Ismaili, J., Urbain, J., Gottlieb, P., Brown, A., Hasemann, C.A., Capra, J.D., Meek, K. (1993). Molecular characterization of monoclonal CRIA-positive anti-arsonate antibodies derived from idiotype-negative mice bearing a light chain polymorphism. *Proc. Natl. Acad. Sci. USA* **90**, 9508–12.

83. Mertens, F., Berek, C., Andris, F., Willems, F., Brait, M., Miller, R., Riblet, R.J., Slaoui, M., and Urbain, J. (1990). A private idiotype can become recurrent through genetic recombination and gene(s) unlinked to the Igh locus governs its expression. *Eur. J. Immunol.* **20**, 1815–23.

84. Vora, K.A., and Manser, T. (1985). Altering the antibody repertoire via transgene homologous recombination: evidence for global and clone-autonomous regulation of antigen-driven B cell differentiation. *J. Exp. Med.* **181**, 271–81.

85. Ryelandt, M. De Wit D., Baz, A., Vansanten, G., Huez, F., Nisol, F., Macedo-Soares, F., Barcy, S., Brait, M., Latinne, D., Bazin, H., and Urbain, J. (1995). The perinatal presence of antigen (p-azophenyl-arsonate)/or anti-mu antibodies lead to the loss of the recurrent idiotype (CRI$_A$) in A/J mice. *Int. Immunol.* **7**, 645–52.

86. Willems, F., Vansanten-Urbain, G., De Wit, D., Slaoui, M., and Urbain, J. (1990). Loss of a major idiotype (CRIA) after repopulation of irradiated mice. *J. Immunol.* **144**, 1396–403.

87. Brait, M., Ryelandt, M., Ismaili, J., Miller, R., Vansanten, G., Riblet, R., and Urbain, J. (1994). Selection of anti-arsonate idiotype (CRIA) in A/J mice by the immune network. *Adv. Exp. Med. Biol.* **355**, 45–9.

88. Ismaili, J., Razanajaona, D., Van Acker, A., Wuilmart, C., Mancini, I., Heinen, E., Leo, O., Lebecque, S., Urbain, J., and Brait, M. (1999). Molecular and cellular basis of the altered immune response against arsonate in irradiated A/J mice autologously reconstituted. *Int. Immunol.* **11**, 1157–67.

89. Linton, P.J.L., Decker, D.J., and Klinman, N.R. (1989). Primary antibody-forming cells and secondary B-cells are generated from separate precursor cell subpopulations. *Cell* **59**, 1049–59.

90. Klinman, N.R. (1998). Repertoire diversification of primary vs memory B cell subsets. *Curr. Top. Microbiol. Immunol.* **229**, 133–48.

91. Decker, D.J., Linton, P.J., Zaharevitz, S., Biery, M., Gingeras, T.R., Klinman, N.R. (1995). Defining subsets of naive and memory B-cells based on the ability of their progeny to somatically mutate in vitro. *Immunity* **2**, 195–203.

92. Gu, H., Tarlinton, D., Muller, W., Rajewsky, K., Forster, I. (1991). Most peripheral B-cells are ligand selected. *J. Exp. Med.* **173**, 1357–1371.

93. Lam, K.P., Kuhn, R., Rajewsky, K. (1997). *In vivo* ablation of surface immunoglobulin on mature B-cells by inducible gene targeting results in rapid cell death. *Cell* **90**, 1073–83.

94. Pillai, S. (1999). The chosen few? Positive selection and the generation of naive B lymphocytes. *Immunity* **10**, 493–502.

95. Lam, K.P., and Rajewsky, K. B. (1999). Cell antigen receptor specificity and surface density together determine B-1 versus B-2 cell development. *J. Exp. Med.* **190**, 471–7.

96. Hayakawa, K., Asano, M., Shinton, S.A., Gui, M., Allman, D., Stewart, C.L., Silver, J., and Hardy, R.R. (1999). Positive selection of natural autoreactive B-cells. *Science* **285**, 113–116.

97. Martin, F., and Kearney, J.F. (2000). B-cell subsets and the mature preimmune repertoire. Marginal zone and B1 B-cells as part of a "natural immune memory". *Immunol. Rev.* **175**, 70–9.

98. Hachemi-Rachedi, S., Drapier, A.M., Cazenave, P.A., and Sanchez, P. (2000). Affiliation to mature B cell repertoire and positive selection can be separated in two distinct processes. *Int. Immunol.* **12**, 385–95.

99. Levine, M.H., Haberman, A.M., Sant'Angelo, D.B., Hannum, L.G., Cancro, M.P., Janeway, C.A. Jr., and Shlomchik, M.J. (2000). A B-cell receptor-specific selection step governs immature to mature B cell differentiation. *Proc. Natl. Acad. Sci. USA* **97**, 2743–8.

100. Cariappa, A., Tang, M., Parng, C., Nebelitskiy, E., Carroll, M., Georgopoulos, K., and Pillai, S. (2001). The Follicular versus Marginal Zone B Lymphocyte Cell Fate Decision Is Regulated by Aiolos, Btk, and CD21. *Immunity* **14**, 603–15.

101. Martin, F., Oliver, A.M., and Kearney, J.F. (2001). Marginal Zone and B1 B-cells Unite in the Early Response against T-Independent Blood-Borne Particulate Antigens. *Immunity* **14**, 617–29.

102. Hilschmann, N., Barnikol, H.U., Barnikol-Watanabe, S., Gotz, H., Kratzin, H., and Thinnes, F.P. (2001). The immunoglobulin-like genetic predetermination of the brain: the protocadherins, blueprint of the neuronal network. *Naturwissenschaften* **88**, 2–12.

103. Crick, F., and Koch, C. (1997). The problem of consciousness. In Mysteries of the mind. *Sc. Am.* 18–29.

104. Damasio, A. (1994). *Descartes Error*. Putman Book, New York.
105. Edelman, G.M., and Tononi, G. (2000). A universe of consciousness : how matter becomes imagination. Basic books.
106. Dennett, D. (1996). Kinds of minds: towards an understanding of consciousness. Weidenfeld and Nicolson, London.
107. Pinker, S. (1997). *How the mind works*. Norton and Company, New York.
108. Greenfield, S. (2000) *The private life of brain*. John Wiley and Sons Inc.
109. Anderson, C.C., Matzinger, and P. Danger (2000).: the view from the bottom of the cliff. *Semin. Immunol.* **12**, 231–8, discussion 257–344.
110. Van Acker, A., Urbain-Vansanten, G., Mariamé, B., Tasiaux, N., De Vos-Cloetens, C., and Urbain, J. (1979). Synthesis of antibodies and immunoglobulins bearing recipient allotypic markers and donor idiotypic specificities in irradiated rabbits grafted with allogeneic cells from hyperimmune donors. *Am. Immunol.* **130C**, 397–406.

Chapter

TWO

The Utility of Immunoglobulin Fusions in DNA Immunization

Alexandra J. Corbett [1,2], Brent S. McKenzie [1,2], Robyn M. Sutherland [1], Jamie L. Brady [1], Richard A. Strugnell [3], Stephen J. Kent [4], David R. Kramer [5], Jeffrey S. Boyle [6], Martin J. Pearse [6] and Andrew M. Lew [1,2]

[1] *The Walter & Eliza Hall Institute of Medical Research and* [2] *CRC for Vaccine Technology, P.O. Royal Melbourne Hospital, Parkville 3050, Australia*
[3] *CRC for Vaccine Technology and Department of Microbiology & Immunology, University of Melbourne, Australia*
[4] *Department of Microbiology & Immunology, University of Melbourne, Australia*
[5] *Centre for Cellular & Molecular Biology, Deakin University, Burwood 3125, Australia*
[6] *CSL Ltd, Parkville 3052, Australia*

I. INTRODUCTION

Most of the currently available vaccines for humans are excellent. We predict that DNA vaccines will not replace the excellent ones with their long history of efficacy and safety. Most of these commercial vaccines (tetanus, diphtheria, pertussis, Hemophilus influenzae B, hepatitis B, measles) probably act via antibody (Ab) mediated mechanisms. Indeed, one can correlate Ab levels with protection for such diseases as measles and tetanus. It is therefore noteworthy that DNA vaccines have been particularly disappointing in eliciting Ab responses in large animals including humans [1–5]. Our laboratory has focused on improving the potency of DNA vaccines and a key feature of this has been the use of immunoglobulin fusions. This review will highlight the utility conferred on such DNA vaccines by the properties of the immunoglobulin moiety.

II. IMMUNOGLOBULIN PROVIDES HELPER DETERMINANTS

Some proteins are poorly immunogenic. The production of Ab can be problematic against tumor neoantigens, allotypic variants, mutant proteins, and proteins which are highly conserved between species. Traditionally, Ab has been raised by immunization with either purified protein or cells expressing the protein of interest. There can be a failure to generate such Ab. The risk of generating Ab of other specificities (e.g., against alloantigens or co-purified proteins other than that being targeted) is high, especially in cases where strong adjuvants are used. Therefore, the specificity of the Ab raised is critically dependent on the purity of the protein. Even minor contaminants can provoke a dominant Ab response [6]. DNA immunization offers the advantage of defined specificity (cloned DNA ensures the absence of other genes), expression of the protein in its native conformation, and derivation of high avidity Ab [7].

Elicitation of Ab to CD45 allotypes is notoriously difficult and previous studies have used allogeneic cell immunizations between mouse strains differing in a number of loci in order to generate anti-CD45 allotype specific Ab [8, 9]. Indeed, cross-immunizations between CD45 congenic mouse strains have proven unsuccessful [9]. We have used DNA encoding Ig fusion molecules for raising Ab against CD45 allotypic variants [10]. The extracellular domains of CD45 were fused to the amino-terminal end of the Fc of human IgG. Immunization with DNA encoding such fusions resulted in increased Ab responses to CD45 allotypes. We believe that like chemical conjugation, genetic fusion with human IgG provided helper determinants. This is because non-responsiveness in mice was overcome by using human Ig but not by using mouse Ig. This concurs with previous work that showed that Ab idiotype proteins were much more immunogenic when engineered to contain foreign constant regions [11].

Others have also shown gene gun immunization with Ig fusions to be effective [12], although direct comparisons of immunogenicity with or without Ig fusions were not made.

We consider that our approach of immunization with DNA encoding the protein of interest fused to the Fc of foreign immunoglobulin should be widely applicable in raising polyclonal or monoclonal Ab specific for other poorly immunogenic proteins. Furthermore, it will be of interest to see if this approach can be applied clinically in increasing responses to poorly immunogenic proteins from pathogens.

III. IMMUNOGLOBULIN INCREASES BIOLOGICAL HALF-LIFE

Many studies have explored the use of cytokines to boost or deviate the immune response. This has entailed either co-injection of plasmids encoding cytokines or plasmids encoding antigen–cytokine fusions. Most have shown only modest effects e.g., 0.1 OD change at a serum dilution of 1:100 when granulocyte-macrophage colony-stimulating factor (GM-CSF) was coinjected, with no effect on the cellular response [13]. Many different cytokines have been tried including IL-2 [14, 15], IL-12 [16, 17], IL-15 [16, 17], IL-18 [18, 19] and MIP-1α [20]. IFN-γ have enhanced responses in some cases [21] and decreased in others [22].

The usefulness of many biological molecules is hindered by their short half-life *in vivo*. Cytokines with half-lives usually of a few minutes provide a poignant example. Bolus doses are precluded for toxicity reasons and any therapeutic regimen requires frequent injections of cytokines. Fortunately, their biological half-lives can be extended by fusing the cytokines to the Fc of IgG. The half-life of IL-2-Ig is 200-fold greater than recombinant IL-2 (25 hr vs 2–9 min respectively) [23]. Whereas IL-15 has a half-life of 2–3 min, IL-15-Ig fusions had a half-life of 6 hr [24]. Similarly, IL-10-Ig fusions increased the half-life of IL-10 from 2 hr [25] to 33 hr [26]. Even more remarkably, TNFR-Ig fusions can have an *in vivo* half-life of 6 days [27].

Genetic delivery of cytokines has the advantage that it avoids the adverse effects of delivering large quantities of protein. IL-12 when delivered as a protein can produce significant non-specific effects. When delivered as a plasmid encoding an antigen fusion, these effects were reduced, whilst maintaining antigen-specific enhancement of responses [16]. In a separate study, no adverse effects of chemokine–antigen fusions over the PBS control were found over a 100-day period in mice immunized with IP-10 or MCP-3 fusions [28]. Although these studies used antigen–cytokine fusions, the same advantage should be afforded to DNA immunization with cytokine–Ig fusions.

The utility of cytokine–Ig fusions in DNA vaccination has been highlighted in a recent HIV model. Rhesus monkeys given DNA vaccines plus IL-2-Ig protein or IL-2-Ig plasmid DNA showed an enhanced cytotoxic T-lymphocyte (CTL) response [15]. Clinical and laboratory (e.g., preservation of CD4 T-cell counts) correlates of protection were superior in the IL-2 augmented vaccinees, whereas the DNA vaccine alone led to modest and heterogeneous outcomes.

In a variant form of DNA immunization, plasmids encoding IFNγR-Ig and IL-4-Ig protected non-obese diabetic (NOD) mice from developing autoimmune diabetes [29].

IV. TARGETING WITH IMMUNOGLOBULIN FUSIONS

Fc Receptor Targeting

Fc receptor (FcR) targeting by antigen–Ig fusions seems to improve the efficiency of antigen presenting cells *in vitro* [30]. There is also the potential to use different IgG subclasses. For example, hIgG3 has the highest affinity for CD64, the high affinity FcγR, and fusions with hIgG3 are superior in activating LAK cells [31].

One group purports an enhancement in DNA vaccination by targeting FcR of dendritic cells *in vivo* by using a fusion molecule of a viral antigen and Fc of human IgG1 [32]. DNA encoding the Fc fusion produced more potent immune responses (Ab, Th and CTL) than DNA encoding the viral antigen alone. Given our above arguments that Ig fusions have many effects including provision of helper epitopes, change of biological half-life and dimerization (discussed below), it is hard to differentiate whether the enhancement is due to these effects rather than to FcR targeting. They argued that the enhancement was FcR-mediated by showing that FcR knockout mice did not respond. However, this was not convincing, as there was no demonstration that the FcR knockout mice could respond to another immunogen that did not have a Fc.

There are further caveats to the interpretation of FcR targeting *in vivo*. There are many types of FcR molecules, including CD64, CD32, CD16 and CD23 [33]. They vary in what cell types they are expressed and in their function. Some have enhancing functions and some have suppressive ones [33]. Therefore, it can be difficult to determine which FcR on which cell is being affected *in vivo*. Nevertheless, the immunogenicity of immune complexes (cf. their tolerogenicity) is generally believed to be due to their binding to FcR on follicular dendritic cells. These cells then present the antigen to B-cells and perhaps also prevent the immune complexes from binding to the inhibitory FcR on B-cells [34]. Any enhancing role of other dendritic cells in seeing the Fc of immune complexes has not been demonstrated.

Ligand Targeting with Ig Fusions

To address the issue of efficacy, we (and others) have previously studied aspects of DNA immunization that may influence the strength and type of immune responses, such as cellular localization of Ag and route of administration [7, 35, 36]. Other approaches (use of immunostimulating sequences, cytokines, costimulator molecules) have had some success in addressing the issue of inducing potent immune responses but have led to relatively minor improvements.

By far the most dramatic effect we have found is the use of a strategy that compensates for the low levels of antigen produced by DNA immunization by delivering the antigen to the sites of immune induction, viz. the secondary lymphoid organs [37]. These organs (spleen, lymph nodes, Peyer's patches etc.) are pivotal in generating immune responses [38]. By delivering antigens to such sites, the antigen level at "where the action is" may be increased. Notably, direct injection into the spleen [39–41] or lymph nodes [42] have been used to augment immune responses. Injections into the organs above are unlikely to be acceptable for routine vaccination. To target antigen to lymphoid sites more practicably, we reasoned that extracellular portions of certain cell surface receptors could act as ligands that bind to or near sites of immune induction. Thus, soluble fusion molecules consisting of antigen and these targeting ligands improve the probability of a small dose of protein being retained or transported to the secondary lymphoid organs. The two ligands chosen were L-selectin and CTLA4. L-selectin binds to CD34 in high endothelial venules of peripheral lymph nodes and CTLA4 to B7 (CD80 and CD86) expressing cells including antigen presenting cells (APCs) which are potent initiators of the immune response. The Fc portion of human IgG1 served not only as the model antigen but as a suitable molecule that survives in the circulation long enough for our targeting strategy to work. Mice were immunized with three DNA constructs: CD5L-hIg (leader sequence of CD5 for secretion of the Fc of human IgG1), Lsel-hIg (leader and extracellular domains of L-selectin N-terminal to the Fc) and CTLA4-hIg (leader and extracellular domains of CTLA4 N-terminal to the Fc). The mature protein expressed by these vectors is schematically illustrated in Figure 1 and the ligand-targeting strategy is outlined in Figure 2.

We found that the immune response to the antigen was dramatically increased [37]. Specific Ab levels in mice were 10,000 fold higher in CTLA4-hIg DNA immunized mice at 2 wks (Figure 3). At 8 wks Ab levels had reached a plateau and were 1000- and 75-fold higher than hIg controls with CTLA4-hIg and Lsel-hIg respectively. Targeting antigen with L-selectin and CTLA4 also enhanced the

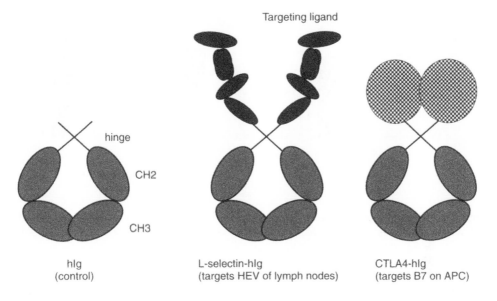

Figure 1. Schematic of the untargeted Fc of human IgG1, L-selectin fusion and CTLA4 fusion proteins.

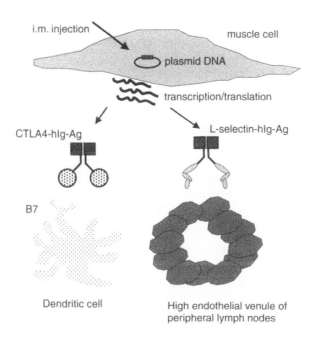

Figure 2. Mammalian expression plasmids encoding antigens fused to targeting ligands. These are injected intramuscularly and the host cell secretes the encoded fusion protein, CTLA4-hIg-antigen or L-selectin-hIg-antigen. CTLA4 targets B7 on antigen presenting cells and L-selectin binds the special carbohydrate groups on CD34 present in high endothelial venule cells of peripheral lymph nodes. Thus the antigen is delivered to lymphoid tissue and hence presented more efficiently. Adapted from [67].

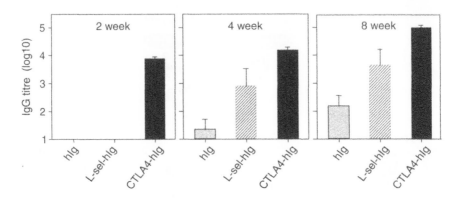

Figure 3. Targeting ligands fused to antigen dramatically enhance the Ab response so that at 8 weeks, there was 100-fold enhancement for L-selectin (L-sel) and 1000-fold for CTLA4.

T-cell proliferative response. Proliferation was increased 2- to 3-fold after Lsel-hIg immunization, whereas up to an 8-fold increase was achieved with CTLA4-hIg. Coinjection of plasmids encoding OVA showed that the CTLA4 had to be fused to the antigen to have an effect and that there was no immunomodulation of OVA responses by the CTLA4-hIg. We were able to confirm the enhancement by CTLA4 with protein immunizations (using proteins purified on protein A from the supernatants of transfected cell lines). Mice that received a single i.m. injection of the soluble CTLA4-Ig protein had significantly higher Ab responses compared to human Ig.

There are several key features of immune responses elicited by the targeting ligands:

1 augmentation of the Ab and CD4 T cell responses;
2 increased speed of the Ab response;
3 predominance of IgG1 with CTLA4 targeting. Most DNA immunizations mimic viral infections in that they elicit IgG2a responses. Levels of certain subclasses may be important in vaccine efficacy [43–46];
4 high number of responding mice with CTLA4 targeting. We have immunized over 100 mice of 3 strains of different H-2 haplotype with CTLA4-hIg and all have produced Abs by 2 wks after injection.

To ascertain the effect of antigen targeting on challenge studies, we have constructed vectors in which a gly-gly-gly-gly-thr spacer was attached to the carboxy-terminus of human IgG1 followed by a multiple cloning site. The IgG component enables dimerization which is critical for the augmentation effect, but can be replaced with other dimerization moieties like the hinge of human IgG3 [47] (discussed below). The multiple cloning site avails the insertion of other antigens C-terminal of our targeting vector. The application of a target-antigen approach has been shown to increase the immune response and enhance protection in infectious and tumor challenge models [5, 48, 49].

Influenza A/Puerto Rico/8/34 H1 (PR8) HA was fused to hIg or CTLA4-hIg (the non-targeted and targeted molecules, respectively). Sephacryl chromatography revealed that the native structures of proteins produced by transfectants were 1.0

and 1.2 million Da in size. We originally thought that these sizes are consistent with higher-ordered structures (e.g., tetramers of dimers: the hIg acting as a dimerization moiety). HA normally forms trimers [50], but higher-order structures may be formed from non-native disulfide bonding or may be predisposed by the juxtaposition of HA by the hIg dimerization. However, the fusion proteins may have a more elongated structure than native HA which gives an aberrantly higher molecular size on molecular sieving so that these molecules may have been trimers of dimers as we would have predicted. Anyway, in the context of this study, what is important is that both targeted and non-targeted molecules oligomerize similarly (the size ratio between subunit and native structure was similar for both), and thus differential oligomerization is not the reason for the enhanced Ab responses with the CTLA4-Ig-HA fusion.

Surprisingly, the majority of the Ab generated by fusion molecules recognized native rather than denatured epitopes. Hemagglutinin has a rather complicated structure and must not have been too constrained by the IgG moiety being fused in front of it.

The targeted DNA vaccine against influenza, CTLA4-Ig-HA generated higher Ab levels ($p < 0.001$; Mann–Whitney) and protected mice by reducing viral titers 100-fold ($p < 0.0004$; Mann–Whitney; Figure 4) compared with the untargeted vaccine. As the CTL responses were not different, this difference in protection was probably Ab based. Incidentally, Ab levels and protection afforded by the targeted vaccine was not significantly different from that afforded by the protein-based commercial split vaccine (Figure 4). However, that this comparison is not germane, because the latter contains neuraminidase components in addition to HA. Moreover, as outlined in the introduction, our strategy aims to improve on currently investigated DNA vaccine strategies through targeting so that they could be used, for example, where no current vaccine exists, rather than as a replacement for effective protein-based (or for that matter live virus) vaccines.

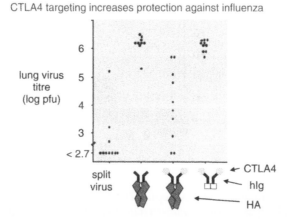

Figure 4. In a challenge model in mice, DNA immunization using CTLA4-ligand targeting induced greater viral (influenza) clearance than that induced by non-targeted DNA immunization.

Importantly targeting via CTLA4 was also employed to overcome the relatively poor efficacy of DNA vaccines in large animals [5]. It was shown that the highest level of protection for the DNA vaccines tested against *Corynebacterium pseudotuberculosis* in sheep was achieved with a first generation CTLA4 fusion vaccine. The vaccine consisted of an antigen (detoxified phospholipase D; PLD) fused to the C-terminus of the human IgG1 heavy chain (hIg to give CTLA4-hIg-PLD). This did not impede the binding to B7 by flow cytometry [5]. Cross-bred ewes aged 12 wks were used in the challenge trial. Any husbandry procedures that could cut the skin (e.g. shearing, tail docking) were avoided to minimize risk of infection with *C. pseudotuberculosis*. Animals were pre-screened for the presence of Ab to PLD and to *C. pseudotuberculosis* lysate. Positive animals were excluded from the trial. Ten animals were allocated randomly to each group. The sheep were immunized with 0.5 mg DNA twice a month and challenged with 10^6 CFU of *C. pseudotuberculosis* injected just above the coronet. Protection was defined as the animal not having abscesses in any of the following lymph nodes: popliteal, inguinal and both left and right prefemoral. The highest degree of protection was observed in the group injected with the targeting vector viz. CTLA4-hIg-PLD (Figure 5).

We believe that the major if not the sole mechanism of this enhancement is anatomical delivery, for several reasons. L-selectin can also be used as a targeting moiety to enhance the immune response to certain antigens [37]; it is difficult to envisage how any signaling to high endothelial venule cells would lead to the enhancement of a specific Ab response. Coinjection of L-selectin-hIg or CTLA4-hIg with ovalbumin does not enhance any responses to ovalbumin [37]; therefore, the effect cannot be a non-specific effect on homing or migration. The B7 cytoplasmic tail is not conserved and has not been shown to signal. Indeed, we have not been able to show, in calcium flux or kinase studies, any effect of CTLA4Ig on B-cells or dendritic cells. In contrast, we have shown preferential localization of the targeted antigen to draining lymph nodes using radioiodinated protein [48]. We

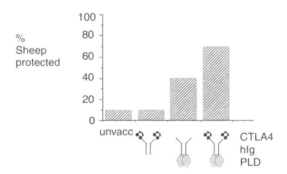

Figure 5. In a large animal model (sheep), CTLA4 targeting with hIg as a dimerization moiety and phospholipase D of *Corynebacterium pseudotuberculosis* is the most effective at protection against challenge. Percentage of the animals protected from challenge by 10^6 CFU of *C. pseudotuberculosis* injected just above the coronet. Protection was defined as the animal not having abscesses in any of the following lymph nodes: popliteal, inguinal and prefemoral both left and right.

therefore contend that physical delivery would seem to be a major, if not the only, mechanism for immune enhancement.

CTLA4-Ig targeting can increase Ab and Th responses, but it neither increases nor decreases CTL responses at least in the two examples we have tested. These were against influenza hemagglutinin (PR8 strain) in H-2^d mice [48] and the ovalbumin CTL epitope SIINFEKL in H-2^b mice [47]. There have been several reports examining the mechanism of CTL induction after intramuscular DNA injection that indicate a role for cross-presentation of antigen [51] via bone marrow derived antigen presenting cells [52–55]. At present, the cross-presenting antigen presenting cell is believed to be a CD8 + dendritic cell [56] and the optimal antigen source is a cell-associated form [57]. Our targeting strategy of a secreted molecule (thus not cell-associated) may not affect these mechanisms of cross-presentation. In any case, DNA injections (e.g., of OVA in mice) already elicit strong CTL responses so that any enhancement in CTL induction by targeting may be difficult to show.

CTLA4 targeting has also been shown for protein immunizations [37, 49]. CTLA4 fused to the C-terminus of a B-cell lymphoma IgG idiotype gave enhanced anti-idiotype Ab and T-cell proliferative responses when compared with untargeted idiotype immunization [49]. When challenged with tumor, the mice given this fusion were better protected. This enhanced immunogenicity was due to B7-binding as anti-idiotype Ab was not enhanced when a mutant CTLA4 that did not bind B7 was used.

Our tenet from these studies is that the dose of antigen given is different from the effective dose. Conventional parenteral immunization will have a more random (wasteful) distribution (this may be inconsequential, when there is excess immunogen). However, the effective dose is what reaches the secondary lymphoid organs and targeting helps to achieve this efficiently and may be critical when antigen is limiting such as in DNA immunization.

V. IMMUNOGLOBIN AS A DIMERIZATION MOIETY

The Fc of IgG dimerizes. Dimerization is important for two major reasons. First, multiple copies of either B-cell epitopes or helper epitopes have been shown to increase immunogenicity [58–62]. Second, multimerization is often required for functional avidity of ligand–receptor binding and not surprisingly, dimerization is required for the enhancement effect of targeting CTLA4-antigen fusions [47] (discussed above). CTLA4-antigen monomers did not enhance Ab responses.

Other dimerization moieties such as leucine zippers could theoretically substitute for IgG. However, for targeting, we argued that the biological half-life of the fusion molecules *in vivo* may be critical and that IgG molecules have been selected by nature to circulate. In some cases, allosteric hindrance by the bulky Fc of IgG can occur. Therefore, if bulkiness is a factor, we chose to substitute the Fc of IgG with the hinge region of human IgG3 (Figure 6). Human IgG3 has an elongated hinge region (about four times longer than human IgG1) with 11 disulphide bonds and hence would be expected to reliably form dimers. This provides a natural spacer and hinge presumably allowing more scope for structural manoeuvring by any antigen fused behind it. In some cases, we have found that the IgG3 hinge fusions with L-selectin as targeting ligand were

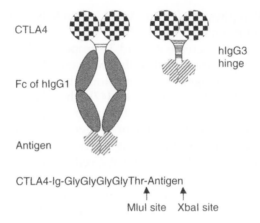

Figure 6. Use of human IgG1 or human IgG3 hinge as dimerization moieties. Schematic of antigens fused to the C-terminus of human IgG1 or human IgG3 hinge; there are two disulphide bonds in the hinge of IgG1 and eleven in IgG3. The fused targeting moiety CTLA4 is also shown.

superior to that of IgG1 Fc fusions. It is interesting that the hinge endows IgG3 with enhanced HIV-neutralizing ability [46].

VI. OTHER FEATURES OF IMMUNOGLOBULIN FUSIONS

Ig fusions also allow the fused antigen to be secreted. This is advantageous in DNA immunization, as we and others have previously found secreted antigen elicited greater Ab responses [35, 63–65]. This occurred whether a naturally non-secreted protein was converted to a secreted one [63, 64] or a naturally secreted protein to membrane bound or cytoplasmic forms [35]. In all these cases, the secreted antigen was the most immunogenic.

Much is known about the Ig isotypes and Fc structure-function relationships so that the Fc can be selected/modified for a chosen purpose. For example, the Fc can be selected from various subclasses depending on the desired property such that an IgG3-IL-2 fusion (which has the extended half-life of 7 hr) has increased binding to FcR on killer cells [66]. The appropriate sites of Fc can also be modified to reduce complement or FcR binding activity [26].

ACKNOWLEDGMENTS

We acknowledge the support of JDRF, NHMRC and CRC-VT.

REFERENCES

1. Calarota, S., Bratt, G., Nordlund, S., Hinkula, J., Leandersson, A. C., Sandstrom, E., and Wahren, B. (1998). Cellular cytotoxic response induced by DNA vaccination in HIV-1- infected patients. *Lancet* **351**, 1320–1325.

2. Wang, R., Doolan, D. L., Le, T. P., Hedstrom, R. C., Coonan, K. M., Charoenvit, Y., Jones, T. R., Hobart, P., Margalith, M., Ng, J., Weiss, W. R., Sedegah, M., de Taisne, C., Norman, J. A., and Hoffman, S. L. (1998). Induction of antigen-specific cytotoxic T lymphocytes in humans by a malaria DNA vaccine. *Science* **282**, 476–480.

3. MacGregor, R. R., Boyer, J. D., Ugen, K. E., Lacy, K. E., Gluckman, S. J., Bagarazzi, M. L., Chattergoon, M. A., Baine, Y., Higgins, T. J., Ciccarelli, R. B., Coney, L. R., Ginsberg, R. S., and Weiner, D. B. (1998). First human trial of a DNA-based vaccine for treatment of human immunodeficiency virus type 1 infection: safety and host response. *J. Infect. Dis.* **178**, 92–100.

4. Babiuk, L. A., Lewis, P. J., Cox, G., van Drunen Littel-van den Hurk, S., Baca-Estrada, M., and Tikoo, S. K. (1995). DNA immunization with bovine herpesvirus-1 genes. *Ann. N Y Acad. Sci.* **772**, 47–63.

5. Chaplin, P. J., De Rose, R., Boyle, J. S., McWaters, P., Kelly, J., Tennent, J. M., Lew, A. M., and Scheerlinck, J. P. (1999). Targeting improves the efficacy of a DNA vaccine against *Corynebacterium pseudotuberculosis* in sheep. *Infect. Immun.* **67**, 6434–6438.

6. Cohn, M., Wetter, L. R., and Deutsch, H. F. (1949). Immunological studies on egg white proteins. I. Precipitation of chicken-ovalbumin and conalbumin by rabbit- and horse-antisera. *J. Immunol.* **61**, 283–296.

7. Boyle, J. S., Silva, A., Brady, J. L., and Lew, A. M. (1997). DNA immunization: induction of higher avidity antibody and effect of route on T cell cytotoxicity. *Proc. Natl. Acad. Sci. USA* **94**, 14626–14631.

8. Shen, F. W., *Monoclonal antibodies to mouse lymphocyte differentiation alloantigens*, Elsevier/North Holland and Biomedical Press, Amsterdam 1981.

9. Scheid, M. P., and Triglia, D. (1979). Further description of the Ly-5 system. *Immunogenetics* **9**, 423–433.

10. Sutherland, R. M., McKenzie, B. S., Corbett, A. J., Brady, J. L., and Lew, A. M. (2001). Overcoming the poor immunogenicity of a protein by DNA immunization as a fusion construct. *Immunol. Cell Biol.* **79**, 49–53.

11. Timmerman, J. M., and Levy, R. (2000). Linkage of foreign carrier protein to a self-tumor antigen enhances the immunogenicity of a pulsed dendritic cell vaccine. *J. Immunol.* **164**, 4797–4803.

12. Kilpatrick, K. E., Cutler, T., Whitehorn, E., Drape, R. J., Macklin, M. D., Witherspoon, S. M., Singer, S., and Hutchins, J. T. (1998). Gene gun delivered DNA-based immunizations mediate rapid production of murine monoclonal antibodies to the Flt-3 receptor. *Hybridoma* **17**, 569–576.

13. Kim, J. J., Bagarazzi, M. L., Trivedi, N., Hu, Y., Kazahaya, K., Wilson, D. M., Ciccarelli, R., Chattergoon, M. A., Dang, K., Mahalingam, S., Chalian, A. A., Agadjanyan, M. G., Boyer, J. D., Wang, B., and Weiner, D. B. (1997). Engineering of *in vivo* immune responses to DNA immunization via codelivery of costimulatory molecule genes. *Nat. Biotechnol.* **15**, 641–646.

14. Bronte, V., Tsung, K., Rao, J. B., Chen, P. W., Wang, M., Rosenberg, S. A., and Restifo, N. P. (1995). IL-2 enhances the function of recombinant poxvirus-based vaccines in the treatment of established pulmonary metastases. *J. Immunol.* **154**, 5282–5292.

15. Barouch, D. H., Santra, S., Schmitz, J. E., Kuroda, M. J., Fu, T. M., Wagner, W., Bilska, M., Craiu, A., Zheng, X. X., Krivulka, G. R., Beaudry, K., Lifton, M. A., Nickerson, C. E., Trigona, W. L., Punt, K., Freed, D. C., Guan, L., Dubey, S., Casimiro, D., Simon, A., Davies, M. E., Chastain, M., Strom, T. B., Gelman, R. S., Montefiori, D. C., and Lewis, M. G. (2000). Control of viremia and prevention of clinical AIDS in rhesus monkeys by cytokine-augmented DNA vaccination. *Science* **290**, 486–492.

16. Kim, J. J., Ayyavoo, V., Bagarazzi, M. L., Chattergoon, M. A., Dang, K., Wang, B., Boyer, J. D., and Weiner, D. B. (1997). *In vivo* engineering of a cellular immune response by coadministration of IL-12 expression vector with a DNA immunogen. *J. Immunol.* **158**, 816–826.

17. Tsuji, T., Hamajima, K., Fukushima, J., Xin, K. Q., Ishii, N., Aoki, I., Ishigatsubo, Y., Tani, K., Kawamoto, S., Nitta, Y., Miyazaki, J., Koff, W. C., Okubo, T., and Okuda, K. (1997). Enhancement of cell-mediated immunity against HIV-1 induced by coinoculation of plasmid-encoded HIV-1 antigen with plasmid expressing IL-12. *J. Immunol.* **158**, 4008–4013.
18. Billaut-Mulot, O., Idziorek, T., Loyens, M., Capron, A., and Bahr, G. M. (2001). Modulation of cellular and humoral immune responses to a multiepitopic HIV-1 DNA vaccine by interleukin-18 DNA immunization/viral protein boost. *Vaccine* **19**, 2803–2811.
19. Maecker, H. T., Hansen, G., Walter, D. M., DeKruyff, R. H., Levy, S., and Umetsu, D. T. (2001). Vaccination with Allergen-IL-18 Fusion DNA Protects Against, and Reverses Established, Airway Hyperreactivity in a Murine Asthma Model. *J. Immunol.* **166**, 959–965.
20. Lu, Y., Xin, K. Q., Hamajima, K., Tsuji, T., Aoki, I., Yang, J., Sasaki, S., Fukushima, J., Yoshimura, T., Toda, S., Okada, E., and Okuda, K. (1999). Macrophage inflammatory protein-1alpha (MIP-1alpha) expression plasmid enhances DNA vaccine-induced immune response against HIV-1. *Clin. Exp. Immunol.* **115**, 335–341.
21. Kim, J. J., Yang, J., Manson, K. H., and Weiner, D. B. (2001). Modulation of antigen-specific cellular immune responses to DNA vaccination in rhesus macaques through the use of IL-2, IFN-gamma, or IL-4 gene adjuvants. *Vaccine* **19**, 2496–2505.
22. Xiang, Z., and Ertl, H. C. (1995). Manipulation of the immune response to a plasmid-encoded viral antigen by coinoculation with plasmids expressing cytokines. *Immunity* **2**, 129–135.
23. Zheng, X. X., Steele, A. W., Hancock, W. W., Kawamoto, K., Li, X. C., Nickerson, P. W., Li, Y., Tian, Y., and Strom, T. B. (1999). IL-2 receptor-targeted cytolytic IL-2/Fc fusion protein treatment blocks diabetogenic autoimmunity in nonobese diabetic mice. *J. Immunol.* **163**, 4041–4048.
24. Kim, Y. S., Maslinski, W., Zheng, X. X., Stevens, A. C., Li, X. C., Tesch, G. H., Kelley, V. R., and Strom, T. B. (1998). Targeting the IL-15 receptor with an antagonist IL-15 mutant/Fc gamma2a protein blocks delayed-type hypersensitivity. *J. Immunol.* **160**, 5742–5748.
25. Li, L., Elliott, J. F., and Mosmann, T. R. (1994). IL-10 inhibits cytokine production, vascular leakage, and swelling during T helper 1 cell-induced delayed-type hypersensitivity. *J. Immunol.* **153**, 3967–3978.
26. Zheng, X. X., Steele, A. W., Nickerson, P. W., Steurer, W., Steiger, J., and Strom, T. B. (1995). Administration of noncytolytic IL-10/Fc in murine models of lipopolysaccharide-induced septic shock and allogeneic islet transplantation. *J. Immunol.* **154**, 5590–5600.
27. Haak-Frendscho, M., Marsters, S. A., Mordenti, J., Brady, S., Gillett, N. A., Chen, S. A., and Ashkenazi, A. (1994). Inhibition of TNF by a TNF receptor immunoadhesin. Comparison to an anti-TNF monoclonal antibody. *J. Immunol.* **152**, 1347–1353.
28. Biragyn, A., Tani, K., Grimm, M. C., Weeks, S., and Kwak, L. W. (1999). Genetic fusion of chemokines to a self tumor antigen induces protective, T-cell dependent antitumor immunity. *Nat. Biotechnol.* **17**, 253–258.
29. Chang, Y., and Prud'homme, G. J. (1999). Intramuscular administration of expression plasmids encoding interferon- gamma receptor/IgG1 or IL-4/IgG1 chimeric proteins protects from autoimmunity. *J. Gene Med.* **1**, 415–423.
30. Durrant, L. G., Parsons, T., Moss, R., Spendlove, I., Carter, G., and Carr, F. (2001). Human anti-idiotypic antibodies can be good immunogens as they target FC receptors on antigen-presenting cells allowing efficient stimulation of both helper and cytotoxic T-cell responses. *Int. J. Cancer* **92**, 414–420.
31. Harvill, E. T., and Morrison, S. L. (1995). An IgG3-IL2 fusion protein activates complement, binds Fc gamma RI, generates LAK activity and shows enhanced binding to the high affinity IL-2R. *Immunotechnology* **1**, 95–105.

32. You, Z., Huang, X., Hester, J., Toh, H. C., and Chen, S. Y. (2001). Targeting dendritic cells to enhance DNA vaccine potency. *Cancer Res.* **61**, 3704–3711.

33. Heyman, B. (2000). Regulation of antibody responses via antibodies, complement, and Fc receptors. *Annu. Rev. Immunol.* **18**, 709–737.

34. Tew, J. G., Wu, J., Fakher, M., Szakal, A. K., and Qin, D. (2001). Follicular dendritic cells: beyond the necessity of T-cell help. *Trends Immunol.* **22**, 361–367.

35. Boyle, J. S., Koniaras, C., and Lew, A. M. (1997). Influence of cellular location of expressed antigen on the efficacy of DNA vaccination: cytotoxic T lymphocyte and antibody responses are suboptimal when antigen is cytoplasmic after intramuscular DNA immunization. *Int. Immunol.* **9**, 1897–1906.

36. Torres, C. A., Iwasaki, A., Barber, B. H., and Robinson, H. L. (1997). Differential dependence on target site tissue for gene gun and intramuscular DNA immunizations. *J. Immunol.* **158**, 4529–4532.

37. Boyle, J. S., Brady, J. L., and Lew, A. M. (1998). Enhanced responses to a DNA vaccine encoding a fusion antigen that is directed to sites of immune induction. *Nature* **392**, 408–411.

38. Karrer, U., Althage, A., Odermatt, B., Roberts, C. W. M., Korsmeyer, S. J., Miyawaki, S., Hengartner, H., and Zinkernagel, R. M. (1997). On the key role of secondary lymphoid organs in antiviral immune responses studied in alymphoplastic (Aly/Aly) and spleenless (Hox11(-/-)) mutant mice. *J. Exp. Med.* **185**, 2157–2170.

39. Gerloni, M., Billetta, R., Xiong, S., and Zanetti, M. (1997). Somatic transgene immunization with DNA encoding an immunoglobulin heavy chain. *DNA Cell Biol.* **16**, 611–625.

40. Boyle, J. S., Barr, I. G., and Lew, A. M. (1999). Strategies for improving responses to DNA vaccines. *Mol. Med.* **5**, 1–8.

41. Moonsom, S., Khunkeawla, P., and Kasinrerk, W. (2001). Production of polyclonal and monoclonal antibodies against CD54 molecules by intrasplenic immunization of plasmid DNA encoding CD54 protein. *Immunol. Lett.* **76**, 25–30.

42. Maloy, K. J., Erdmann, I., Basch, V., Sierro, S., Kramps, T. A., Zinkernagel, R. M., Oehen, S., and Kundig, T. M. (2001). Intralymphatic immunization enhances DNA vaccination. *Proc. Natl. Acad. Sci. USA* **98**, 3299–3303.

43. Beck, O. E. (1981). Distribution of virus antibody activity among human IgG subclasses. *Clin. Exp. Immunol.* **43**, 626–632.

44. Shakib, F. E., *Basic and Clinical Aspects of IgG Subclasses*, Karger, Basel 1986.

45. Snapper, C. M., and Mond, J. J. (1993). Towards a comprehensive view of immunoglobulin class switching. *Immunol. Today* **15**, 15–17.

46. Scharf, O., Golding, H., King, L. R., Eller, N., Frazier, D., Golding, B., and Scott, D. E. (2001). Immunoglobulin G3 from polyclonal human immunodeficiency virus (HIV) immune globulin is more potent than other subclasses in neutralizing HIV type 1. *J. Virol.* **75**, 6558–6565.

47. Lew, A. M., Brady, B. J., and Boyle, B. J. (2000). Site-directed immune responses in DNA vaccines encoding ligand-antigen fusions. *Vaccine* **18**, 1681–1685.

48. Deliyannis, G., Boyle, J. S., Brady, J. L., Brown, L. E., and Lew, A. M. (2000). A fusion DNA vaccine that targets antigen-presenting cells increases protection from viral challenge. *Proc. Natl. Acad. Sci. USA* **97**, 6676–6680.

49. Huang, T. H., Wu, P. Y., Lee, C. N., Huang, H. I., Hsieh, S. L., Kung, J., and Tao, M. H. (2000). Enhanced antitumor immunity by fusion of CTLA-4 to a self tumor antigen. *Blood* **96**, 3663–3670.

50. Wiley, D. C., and Skehel, J. J. (1987). The structure and function of the hemagglutinin membrane glycoprotein of influenza virus. *Annu. Rev. Biochem.* **56**, 365–394.

51. Heath, W. R., and Carbone, F. R. (2001). Cross-presentation, dendritic cells, tolerance and immunity. *Annu. Rev. Immunol.* **19**, 47–64.

52. Doe, B., Selby, M., Barnett, S., Baenziger, J., and Walker, C. M. (1996). Induction of cytotoxic T lymphocytes by intramuscular immunization with plasmid DNA is facilitated by bone marrow derived cells. *Proc. Natl. Acad. Sci.* **93**, 8578.

53. Corr, M., von Damm, A., Lee, D. J., and Tighe, H. (1999). *In vivo* priming by DNA injection occurs predominantly by antigen transfer. *J. Immunol.* **163**, 4721–4727.

54. Iwasaki, A., Torres, C. A., Ohashi, P. S., Robinson, H. L., and Barber, B. H. (1997). The dominant role of bone marrow-derived cells in CTL induction following plasmid DNA immunization at different sites. *J. Immunol.* **159**, 11–14.

55. Ulmer, J. B., Deck, R. R., Dewitt, C. M., Donnhly, J. I., and Liu, M. A. (1996). Generation of MHC class I-restricted cytotoxic T lymphocytes by expression of a viral protein in muscle cells: antigen presentation by non-muscle cells. *Immunology* **89**, 59–67.

56. den Haan, J. M., Lehar, S. M., and Bevan, M. J. (2000). CD8(+) but not CD8(–) dendritic cells cross-prime cytotoxic T cells *in vivo*. *J. Exp. Med.* **192**, 1685–1696.

57. Li, M., Davey, G. M., Sutherland, R. M., Kurts, C., Lew, A. M., Hirst, C., Carbone, F. R., and Heath, W. R. (2001). Cell-associated ovalbumin is cross-presented much more efficiently than soluble ovalbumin *in vivo*. *J. Immunol.* **166**, 6099–6103.

58. Le, T. P., Church, L. W., Corradin, G., Hunter, R. L., Charoenvit, Y., Wang, R., de la Vega, P., Sacci, J., Ballou, W. R., Kolodny, N., Kitov, S., Glenn, G. M., Richards, R. L., Alving, C. R., and Hoffman, S. L. (1998). Immunogenicity of *Plasmodium falciparum* circumsporozoite protein multiple antigen peptide vaccine formulated with different adjuvants. *Vaccine* **16**, 305–312.

59. Kjerrulf, M., Lowenadler, B., Svanholm, C., and Lycke, N. (1997). Tandem repeats of T helper epitopes enhance immunogenicity of fusion proteins by promoting processing and presentation. *Mol. Immunol.* **34**, 599–608.

60. Khan, C. M., Villarreal-Ramos, B., Pierce, R. J., Demarco de Hormaeche, R., McNeill, H., Ali, T., Chatfield, S., Capron, A., Dougan, G., and Hormaeche, C. E. (1994). Construction, expression, and immunogenicity of multiple tandem copies of the Schistosoma mansoni peptide 115–131 of the P28 glutathione S-transferase expressed as C-terminal fusions to tetanus toxin fragment C in a live aro-attenuated vaccine strain of Salmonella. *J. Immunol.* **153**, 5634–5642.

61. Lowenadler, B., Svennerholm, A. M., Gidlund, M., Holmgren, E., Krook, K., Svanholm, C., Ulff, S., and Josephson, S. (1990). Enhanced immunogenicity of recombinant peptide fusions containing multiple copies of a heterologous T helper epitope. *Eur. J. Immunol.* **20**, 1541–1545.

62. Drew, D. R., Boyle, J. S., Lew, A. M., Lightowlers, M. W., and Strugnell, R. A. (2001). The human IgG3 hinge mediates the formation of antigen dimers that enhance humoral immune responses to DNA immunisation. *Vaccine* **19**, 4115–4120.

63. Inchauspe, G., Vitvitski, L., Major, M. E., Jung, G., Spengler, U., Maisonnas, M., and Trepo, C. (1997). Plasmid DNA expressing a secreted or a nonsecreted form of hepatitis C virus nucleocapsid: comparative studies of antibody and T-helper responses following genetic immunization. *DNA Cell Biol.* **16**, 185–195.

64. Svanholm, C., Bandholtz, L., Lobell, A., and Wigzell, H. (1999). Enhancement of antibody responses by DNA immunization using expression vectors mediating efficient antigen secretion. *J. Immunol. Methods* **228**, 121–130.

65. Bucht, G., Sjolander, K. B., Eriksson, S., Lindgren, L., Lundkvist, A., and Elgh, F. (2001). Modifying the cellular transport of DNA-based vaccines alters the immune response to hantavirus nucleocapsid protein. *Vaccine* **19**, 3820–3829.

66. Harvill, E. T., Fleming, J. M., and Morrison, S. L. (1996). *In vivo* properties of an IgG3-IL-2 fusion protein. A general strategy for immune potentiation. *J. Immunol.* **157**, 3165–3170.

67. Langermann, S. (1998). Site-directed immunogenesis. *Nat. Med.* **4**, 547–548.

Chapter

THREE

Constraints on the Hydropathicity and Sequence Composition of HCDR3 are Conserved Across Evolution

Ivaylo Ivanov,[1] Jason Link,[1] Gregory C. Ippolito,[1] and Harry W. Schroeder, Jr.[2]

[1] *Division of Developmental and Clinical Immunology, Department of Microbiology, University of Alabama at Birmingham, Birmingham, Alabama 35294–3300, USA*

[2] *Division of Developmental and Clinical Immunology. Departments of Microbiology and Medicine, University of Alabama at Birmingham, Birmingham, Alabama 35294–3300, USA*

Despite an almost unlimited potential for diversity in the third complementarity determining region of the immunoglobulin H chain (HCDR3), the HCDR3 repertoire that is actually expressed by the adult demonstrates significant constraints. The repertoire of antigen receptors on those B-cells that manage to survive and reach the mature B cell stage is enriched for HCDR3 regions with certain characteristic features, such as a preferred range of hydropathicities and use of a preferred subset of amino acids. These preferences are not unique to mouse or human, but are found in species as diverse as cartilaginous fishes, reptiles, and amphibians. In this review, the mechanisms that act to constrain the HCDR3 component of the antibody repertoire are examined.

Address correspondence to: Dr Harry W. Schroeder, Jr., Division of Developmental and Clinical Immunology, Wallace Tumor Institute 378, 1530 3rd Ave S, University of Alabama at Birmingham, Birmingham, Alabama 35294. Tel: (205) 934–1522; Fax: (205) 975–6352; e-mail: *Harry.Schroeder@ccc.uab.edu*.

I. INTRODUCTION

The capacity of the immune system to recognize a vast array of antigens and distinguish self from non-self depends largely on the ability to generate a diverse, yet balanced, repertoire of antigen-binding receptors. The mechanisms that enhance, as well as those that constrain, antigen–receptor diversity are thus of a fundamental interest.

Among immunoglobulins, diversity is concentrated in the six complementarity determining regions (CDRs) of the heavy and light chains. Amid these CDRs, the third CDR of the heavy (H) chain (HCDR3) is the major focus of diversification of the B-cell pre-immune repertoire (reviewed in [1]). Structurally, HCDR3 lies at the center of the classic antigen-binding site and typically plays a critical role in defining the antigen specificity of the antibody (Figure 1). Genetically, HCDR3 parallels the diversity of the antibody repertoire since it is the direct product of V_H–D_H–J_H recombination (Figure 1B) [2–5]. It is the only region of the antibody encoded by sequence from all three types of germline gene segments. Moreover, mechanisms unique to this immunoglobulin interval, such as the addition of templated (P) and nontemplated (N) nucleotides and the random loss of nucleotides at the joins, provide further means of diversification (reviewed in [6–8]). Thus, the centrally positioned HCDR3 is designed to be the most variable portion of the antibody.

Nevertheless, there is evidence that limitations are imposed even on this region of diversity, such that antigen-binding sites with certain characteristics are preferentially produced. Immunoglobulins containing HCDR3s with neutral or slightly hydrophilic amino acids are preferred in most organisms investigated to date, whereas those that contain HCDR3s with highly charged or hydrophobic sequences are rare or absent. The preference for neutral, hydrophilic sequence begins in the germline. The vast majority of D_H gene segments, which encode

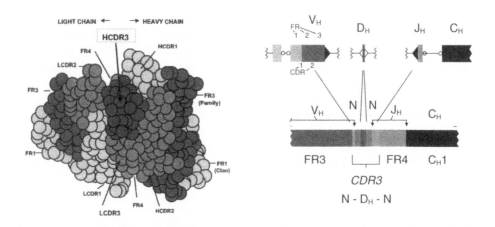

Figure 1. Location and generation of HCDR3. (A) A cartoon of the classic antigen binding site as seen head-on illustrates the central location of HCDR3. (B). HCDR3 is created by VDJ joining and N addition (reviewed in [2]). By virtue of the mechanisms that create it and the position it occupies, HCDR3 is the key to the diversification of the pre-immune repertoire. (See Color plate 1)

much of each HCDR3 sequence, exhibit a characteristic hydropathicity signature for each of their six potential reading frames. Of these six reading frame sequences, only one is typically enriched for the presence of tyrosine and glycine residues, and this is the one that is greatly preferred. Similarly, the JH portion of HCDR3 is typically enriched for neutral, hydrophilic sequence. Thus, although HCDR3 diversity is great, it appears to operate within constraints that are built into the system from the onset of B cell development. The details, as well as potential explanations for these constraints, are discussed below.

II. CONSTRAINTS ON IMMUNOGLOBULIN DIVERSITY

The presence of constraints on the germline diversity of immunoglobulin variable domains was first noted as a result of a cross-species analysis of V gene segment sequence. V gene segments in shark, mouse, and human were found to share extensive sequence homology [1, 9]. The extent of this sequence conservation exceeded that of the constant regions that specify effector function. The V gene segment sequence conservation was shown to have structural correlates, which also help explain why the conservation is not equally distributed across the sequence as a whole. The primary sequence of an Ig V domain is typically subdivided into three highly variable intervals, the complementarity determining regions, or CDRs; and four relatively invariant intervals, termed framework regions (FRs). At the secondary and tertiary structural level, it can be seen that FRs 2 and 4 of the H and L chains unite to form the hydrophobic core of the fragment of an antibody (Fab). FR1 connects the constant domain to the variable domain and forms the external bottom surface of the Fab portion of the antibody. FR3 lies between FR1 and CDRs 1 and 2 and rests on FR2 and 4. It is these framework regions that are primarily conserved across evolution and within V gene families. Given that the frameworks create the foundation upon which the antigen-binding site must rest, the conservation of these regions has thus been attributed to preservation of especially effective backbone. This simple explanation for the conservation of the scaffolds appears intuitively obvious.

What is harder to explain is the conservation of sequence in regions of diversity that are devoted to binding antigen. This is especially intriguing with regard to HCDR3, the predicted focus of diversification, which is presumed to be the *raison d'etre* for immunoglobulins.

Although at first glance the sequence composition of HCDR3 appears random, a closer inspection reveals a number of constraints. First, the sequence composition of the germline-encoded portion of HCDR3 has limited diversity, which again has been conserved across evolution. Certain amino acids, e.g., Tyr and Gly, are overutilized in the germline sequence of diversity (DH) and joining (JH) gene segments, whereas other amino acids, e.g., Arg and Lys, are underutilized. This, together with a skewed reading frame (RF) utilization, helps reduce the range of hydropathicity observed in HCDR3 sequences. Moreover, a variety of selection mechanisms (see below) appear to further reinforce limitations on the range of hydropathicity within HCDR3.

Second, the range of structures available to HCDR3 appears to be constrained. Others and we have shown that the average length of HCDR3 is tightly regulated in human and a number of other organisms [10–12]. The constraints on

HCDR3 length do not seem to depend on the length of the D or J segment that is being used, and it appears as though all diversification mechanisms (P and N addition, exonucleolytic nibbling, etc.) act in concert in this regulation [10].

Finally, the constraints on the composition of HCDR3 appear to be differentially regulated during ontogeny (reviewed in [13–15]). Both molecular mechanisms, such as absence of N regions in the fetus, and antigen receptor-influenced selection – i.e., utilization preference for certain germline segments, lead to the production of a rather different repertoire of Ag receptors in fetus when compared to the repertoire expressed by the adult. Limitations in immune responses of infants have been attributed, at least in part, to these restrictions [16–17].

All of the above features of regulation of the HCDR3 are the subject of intensive investigation by a number of laboratories [10, 12, 18–24]. This review will focus on the nature and the consequences of the constraints on hydropathicity that are imposed, in part, by control of DH reading frame usage.

HYDROPATHICITY AND THE SEQUENCE COMPOSITION OF HCDR3

The hydropathicity of a protein sequence reflects its behavior in an aqueous solution and can be used to predict the nature of its interactions with the external environment and within the structure of the protein itself. In general, hydrophilic side-chains will be soluble in water and will be allowed access to the aqueous solvent, whereas hydrophobic side-chains will tend to be shielded from the water molecules and are more soluble in organic solvents. Charged amino acids are not only highly soluble in aqueous solutions, but they can engage in building salt bridges with amino acids with a complementary charge. Hydropathicity (or hydrophobicity) scales for amino acid residues are a means by which numeric hydropathicity values can be assigned to each amino acid, and thus provide a standard by which the hydropathicity of a series of amino acids can be compared. Different scales utilize different methods for measuring or calculating the hydropathicity values. The methods are based on measurements of free energy of transfer between different solvents or states (water-to-vapor) or from distribution of amino acids in proteins with a known conformation (for a review on different hydropathicity scales see [25, 26]).

We used the Kyte–Doolitle hydropathicity index [27] (Figure 2) to calculate the hydropathicity distribution of HCDR3s from previously published VDJ sequences of several different species (Figure 3). In this index as normalized by Eisenberg [25], the hydropathicity of the various amino acids ranges from a +1.7 for isoleucine, to 0.03 for glycine, to −1.4 for arginine. The average hydropathicity was calculated by adding the hydropathicity value for each amino acid within HCDR3, and then dividing by the number of amino acids.

The range and pattern of HCDR3 hydropathicities was remarkably similar among published sequences of the three species examined – human [24], mouse [28] and shark [29] – in spite of the fact that they belong to widely divergent groups and exist in remarkably different environments. In all three species, a preference for neutral or slightly hydrophilic HCDR3s is observed and highly charged or hydrophobic sequences are rare or absent. Thus, the hydropathicity of HCDR3 appears to be tightly constrained. In order to assess the extent to which these constraints reflect regulation at the genetic level, we examined the sequence

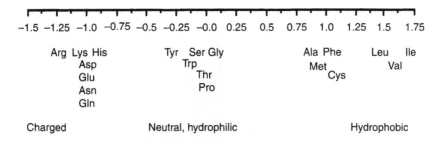

Figure 2. The relative hydropathicity of any given protein sequence can be calculated through use of the Kyte–Doolittle Hydropathicity Index. Kyte and Doolittle assigned hydropathicity values to each amino acid [27]. This scale is used in its normalized form [25] and is represented schematically above. The amino acids are clustered into a charged group, e.g. Arginine at −1.3; a neutral hydrophilic group, e.g., Serine at −0.10; and a hydrophobic group, e.g., Isoleucine at +1.7. The hydropathicity of a protein region (e.g., HCDR3) as a whole can then be determined by calculating the average hydropathicity index value for the amino acid content of the region, e.g., the mouse D segment DFL16.1 encodes the sequence YYYGSSY in reading frame 1. It contains 4 tyrosines – hydropathicity value −0.27, 2 serines – h. value −0.10 and a glycine residue, which carries a hydropathicity value of +0.03. The calculated hydropathicity for this sequence is: −0.18.

composition and hydropathicity of the two germline segments that encode most of HCDR3 – DH and JH – in mouse and human.

DH Gene Segments

The DH gene segment forms the core of HCDR3; thus any limits on the diversity of DH sequence can have a profound influence on the diversity of the antibody repertoire as a whole [30]. It is remarkable, therefore, that in spite of the fact that the D in DH stands for diversity, its sequence composition is actually conserved across evolution.

DH gene segments are small and typically encode fewer than 11 amino acids of the final V domain sequence, all of which are near the carboxyl terminus of the domain [10]. During VDJ recombination, the site of joining between a DH and a JH can vary, with both addition and deletion of nucleotides at the termini [6]. As a result, every D segment has the potential to be joined, transcribed, and translated in any one of three reading frames (RFs) by deletion or three RFs by inversion, and still yield functional sequence. Thus, each D gene segment represents six potential core HCDR3 sequences.

Although the precise sequence of an individual DH gene segment may vary within or between species, the sequence composition of each DH reading frame tends to be non-random and tends to follow a pattern that has been conserved from shark to human. In all species, one of the reading frames by deletion is typically enriched for tyrosine, glycine and serine. In the mouse, this reading frame is used in more than 90% of rearrangements [28] and was thus defined as Reading Frame 1. In this work, the designation RF1, has been extended to all species on the basis of enrichment for these amino acid residues. RF2, which in the mouse generates a Dμ protein, is enriched for hydrophobic amino acid residues, and RF3 is

Shark

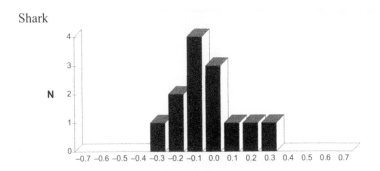

Mouse

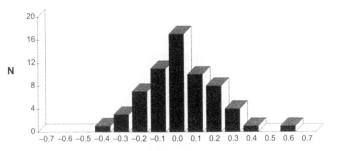

Human

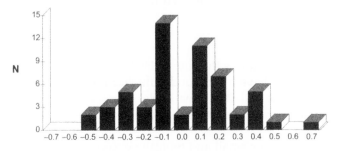

HCDR3 Hydropathicity

Figure 3. Hydropathicity of HCDR3. Shown are average hydropathicities for HCDR3 intervals from randomly cloned VDJ sequences of shark [29], mouse [28], and human [24]. The Gaussian distribution is striking and centered in the neutral, hydrophilic range which characterizes reading frame 1 in all three species (Table 1).

the reading frame that contains termination codons. RF3 also typically contains hydrophobic amino acids, sometimes even more than RF2. The reading frames by inversion (iRFs), exhibit characteristic hydropathicities as well. iRF1 typically contains charged amino acids, whereas the hydropathicities of iRF2 and iRF3 parallel the hydropathicities of their corresponding reading frames by deletion (iRF2 is hydrophobic and iRF3 contains termination codons). The hydropathicities of the 6 RFs of some of the most highly used D segments from three species are shown in Table 1.

Table 1 Amino Acid Sequences of Each of the Six Reading Frames for the D_H1 from *Heterodontus* [29], DFL16.1 from Mouse [54], and D3–22 from Human [22]

Gene segment and reading frame (RF)	Shark		Mouse		Human	
	DH1	Average hydropathicity	DFL16.1	Average hydropathicity	D3–22	Average hydropathicity
RF by deletion						
RF1 (hydrophilic)	*YYSGY*	*−0.18*	*YYYGSSY*	*−0.18*	*YYYDSSGYYY*	*−0.28*
RF2 (hydrophobic)	VLNWV	0.69	FITTVVA	0.95	ITMIVVIT	1.17
RF3 (hydrophobic and termination)	GTTVG	0.30	LLLR**L	0.86	VLL***WLLL	1.18
RF by inversion						
i-RF1 (charged)	THCST	−0.03	SYYRSNK	−0.59	SNNHYYHSN	−0.57
i-RF2 (hydrophobic)	IPTVV	0.96	VATTVVI	1.02	VVITTIIVI	1.08
i-RF3 (hydrophobic and termination)	YPL*Y	0.21	*LLP***	0.92	***PLLS**Y	0.67

The average hydropathicity of each reading frame has been calculated as described below. In all three species, one reading frame is employed preferentially (RF1 by deletion) such that the HCDR3 is conserved to be slightly hydrophilic and enriched for aromatic amino acids [54].

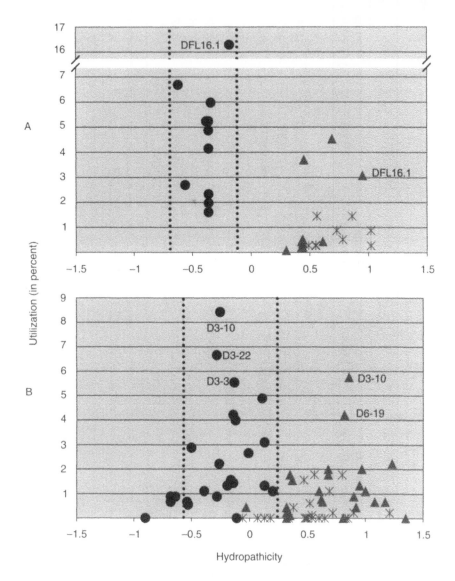

Figure 4. Utilization of reading frames in mouse (A) and human (B) D segments. Each point on the graph represents a germ-line D segment in RF1 (●), RF2 (▲) or RF3 (✳). The hydropathicity of the germline sequence is plotted against the utilization of that sequence in adult VDJ joins. The over-representation of RF1 is obvious in both species. Data used for the calculation of the utilization: mouse – from [28], for human – from [22]. Mouse DQ52 and human D7-27 were not included in the analysis (see text).

This characteristic pattern of hydropathicity by reading frame is well illustrated in the mouse, with virtually every D$_H$ gene segment exhibiting a similar hydropathicity by reading frame (Figure 4A). The only exception is DQ52, which is limited by sequence to a mere 3 codons that are all relatively neutral in hydropathicity. In human, there is somewhat greater variation in hydropathicity between D$_H$ gene segments (i.e., RF1 in D1 and D2 families), but the general characteristics of each reading frame are still the same (Figure 4B). Indeed, the average hydropathicities by reading frame for all the DH gene segments are surprisingly similar to those in mouse (−0.4 for RF1 in mouse and −0.3 for the corresponding reading frame in human).

Because of these conserved patterns in each RF, any limitation in RF usage will lead to constraints in the composition of HCDR3. Indeed, RF preference has been described in almost all species investigated to date. As mentioned above, RF1 is highly preferred in the mouse. It is also used in more than 60% of human adult VDJ joins [21, 22].

There are a variety of mechanisms that can be used to skew reading frame usage and thus bias the amino acid composition of HCDR3.

A preference for DH rearrangement by deletion is one such mechanism. In mouse, for example, the ratio of deletion to inversion has been calculated to be approximately 2000:1 in DJ joins [31]. In human, inverted D elements are also under-represented in the expressed repertoire [22]. This preference for deletion, which is observed in most species, promotes the use of the three corresponding RFs.

The presence of termination codons in RF3 is another common mechanism limiting use of one of the three deletional reading frames. Termination codons are found in RF3 in most mouse and human DH gene segments.

In the mouse, use of RF1 is further promoted by the presence of an upstream ATG translation start site that is in-frame with RF2. Rearrangement in RF2 leads to the production of a Dμ protein that lacks a complete V region but can still activate mechanisms of allelic exclusion, preventing the RF2 expressing B cell progenitor from generating a functional receptor [32]. This mechanism does not appear to operate in human [21].

Finally, early in mouse ontogeny, when N region addition is lacking, sequence identity between the 3′ terminus of DH in RF1 and the 5′ terminus of JH prejudices rearrangement into RF1 [28, 51]. This mechanism also does not appear to operate in human [21]. However, in spite of the fact that the latter two mechanisms are not utilized, the end result is the same, a preference for use of RF1 (Figure 4B).

Non-random usage of RFs with conserved amino acid composition would be presumed to contribute to the non-random amino acid composition of HCDR3. Still the question remains how much of this composition is predetermined in the germline. To elucidate such questions, representation of amino acids in all three deletional RFs of the germline D segments was calculated (second column on Figure 5.1). It was compared to the representation of amino acids in the total expressed proteins for the corresponding organism (first column on Figure 5.1 [33]). Since non-random use of individual DH gene segments further contributes to limitations in the sequence composition of HCDR3, a third analysis was done by normalizing amino acid utilization as a function of DH usage in expressed HCDR3s and as a function of reading frame utilization (third column on Figure 5.1). In this last analysis, a coefficient of utilization was determined for each amino acid encoded by the germline sequence of the D locus. For example, mouse DH DFL16.1 is utilized in ~20% of adult VDJ sequences in mouse and ~80% of these DFL16.1 sequences are in RF1. In contrast, mouse DH DSP2.2 is used only ~7% of the time and only ~30% of the DSP2.2 sequences are in RF1. A Tyr residue in RF1 of DFL16.1 thus achieved a larger coefficient ($0.8 \times 0.2 = 0.16$) than a Tyr residue

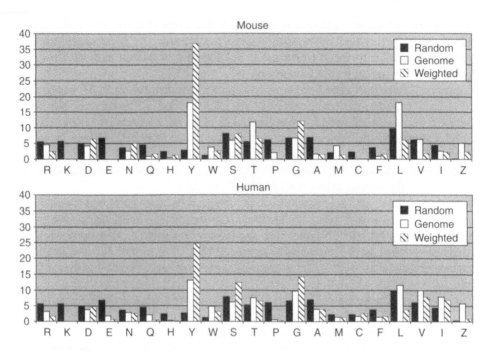

Figure 5.1. Amino acid representation in the three deletional reading frames in mouse and human D segments. The first column for each amino acid corresponds to that amino acid's frequency of occurence (in percent) in all available Genbank protein sequences for that organism [33]. The second column shows the amino acid content of the germline sequence of the D segments (in all three RFs). The third column is the amino acid representation in the D segments weighted according to the usage of each D segment and each reading frame in adult VDJ joins. Z = Stop codons. Data for the calculations from [22, 28].

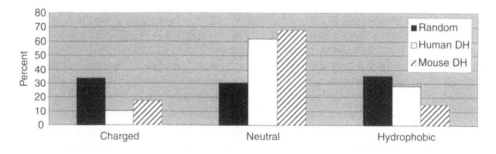

Figure 5.2. Representation of the three groups of amino acids encoded in the human and mouse D segments normalized according to D segment and RF usage as on Figure 5.1 (column 3) and compared to the random representation (first column on Figure 5.1).
Charged aa: R, K, D, E, N, Q, H
Neutral aa: Y, W, S, T, P, G
Hydrophobic aa: A, M, C, F, L, V, I
The random representation is almost identical for both species and only mouse is shown.

in RF1 of DSP2.2 ($0.07 \times 0.3 = 0.021$). The utilization of Tyr was determined from the sum of the number of Tyr residues in each RF in each D segment multiplied by the corresponding coefficients. The values for D segment and RF usage were taken or calculated from the literature – [28] for mouse and [22] for human.

Tyrosine was the only amino acid that was considerably over-represented in both the genomic sequence of the D locus and the normalized analysis. For both organisms the genomic sequence contains 5- to 7-fold more tyrosine compared to the average protein (compare first to the second column on Figure 5.1) and this preference is increased to more than 10-fold when the D segment and RF usage is taken into account (third column). This means that the preference for tyrosine has been predetermined in the germ line and is further augmented by processes of preferential gene rearrangement as well as antigen receptor-influenced selection. The hydropathicity value for Tyr is -0.27, placing it in the slightly hydrophilic range. Other neutral aminoacids like glycine (in both species) and serine (in human) are not over-represented in the germ line sequence but their representation is increased by preferential usage of D segments and/or RFs.

Conversely, charged amino acids are significantly under-represented in both species even at the genomic level. Charged amino acids are two-fold less common in the mouse germline D_H sequences and three-fold less common in the human D_H sequence, when compared to their representation among protein sequences as a whole (Figure 5.2). In the mouse, none of the germline D segments encodes any of the codons for glutamate or lysine in a deletional reading frame. Lysine can only be encoded by the first three nucleotides of DFL16.1 when it is used in an inversional rearrangement. Not only is a rearrangement by inversion a rare event, but due to the process of exonucleolytic nibbling, at least one nucleotide is commonly removed from the 5' end of the D-segment. Thus de facto lysine residue is likely to only appear in HCDR3 as a product of N-region addition. The same is more or less true for glutamate, which can only be encoded by the first three nucleotides of DFL16.2 (again in an inverted reading frame) or in an inverted reading frame of the rarely utilized DST4 gene segment that in addition contains a termination codon.

Hydrophobic amino acids are also much less frequently used, especially in the mouse. It is interesting that this is achieved in a completely different way than the limitations on the other types of amino acids. The hydrophobic residues are actually over-represented in the genomic sequence of both species, mainly because of the characteristics of RF2. But their representation in the repertoire is reduced as a result of differential D segment and RF usage. For example, leucine is twice as common in the germline sequence of the mouse D segments compared to the average mouse protein (column 2 for L on Figure 5.1), but it is actually under-represented in the weighted sum (column 3 for L on Figure 5.1) and hence in the final HCDR3 sequence.

In summary, the over-representation of neutral amino acids and the under-representation of charged residues begins in the germline sequence and is further accentuated with preferential D segment and RF usage. In contrast, the potential for encoding hydrophobic aminoacids in the genomic sequence of the D's is higher than the average peptide sequence, but it is reduced as a result of the same mechanisms listed above, so that those aminoacids will be unlikely to make it into the final repertoire.

The non-random use of amino acids by reading frame is a feature of the germ-line DH repertoire that has been conserved from shark to human. The preferential use of only one of the six potential DH reading frames also appears to be a conserved feature. The driving force behind this conservation remains unclear. Because the DH gene segment forms the core of HCDR3, non-random representation of amino acids coupled with preferential use of a single reading frame serve to limit the final diversity of the antibody repertoire, but whether the pressure to limit the repertoire reflects selection for the generation of beneficial antigen binding sites or selection against generation of non-functional or deleterious antigen binding sites has yet to be definitively addressed. These issues are discussed more fully in a later section of this review.

JH Gene Segments

JH gene segment sequence contributes significantly to HCDR3, providing on average about one-fifth of the amino acids of the interval, all of which are located at the carboxyl terminus [10]. Only the amino terminus of the JH segment is found in HCDR3 – the residues up to, but not including, the conserved Trp at amino acid position 103 (Trp103). The sequence composition and hydropathicity profile of this portion of JH also appears to be non-random. The HCDR3 portion of mouse and human germ line JH gene segments serve to illustrate this pattern (Figure 6A). In general, JH HCDR3 sequence is neutral or slightly hydrophilic, just like DH RF1. For example, all but one JH gene segment in mouse and human have hydropathicity values ranging between -0.23 to $+0.23$. The single exception to this rule is JH3 in both species (Figure 6). The paucity of highly charged or hydrophobic amino acids in JH amino terminal sequence likely contributes to their under-representation in the final HCDR3 structure. Intriguingly, in the human there is a subtle shift in the hydropathicity of the JH portion of HCDR3 as a function of ontogeny. In the fetus, there is preferential use of the more hydrophobic JH gene segments (JH2, 3 and 4), whereas the more neutral or slightly hydrophilic JHs are preferred in the adult (JH4, 5 and 6) [21] (Figure 6B).

In keeping with the pattern observed in DH gene segments, Tyr is the most highly used amino acid in JH gene segments, with more than 50% representation in the sequence before the conserved Phe100 in both species. This preference for Tyr residues reaches an extreme in the second most highly used JH segment in the adult human – JH6, which contains a stretch of 5 Tyr residues at the amino terminus (Figure 6). The presence of a JH gene segment enriched at its amino terminus for Tyrosine residues seems to be a common feature of the germline repertoire in most species (see below).

N Region Addition and other Mechanisms that can Adjust HCDR3 Hydropathicity

Although the mechanisms of recombination that direct reading frame usage appear to strongly prejudice the repertoire towards a germline encoded, neutral, hydrophilic range; even when other reading frames are used, N region addition and exonucleolytic nibbling of DH sequence are a mechanism by which hydropathicity can be adjusted. With the added effects of receptor-influenced selection, VDJ joins containing a DH read in a strongly hydrophobic reading frame can be selected for neutral, hydrophilic sequence.

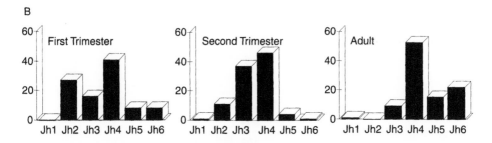

A

J segment	AA Sequence	Hydropathicity
Mouse		
Jh1	Y W Y F D V	0.17
Jh2	Y F D Y	−0.11
Jh3	A W F A Y	0.45
Jh4	Y Y A M D Y	−0.04
Human		
Jh1	A E Y F Q H	−0.22
Jh2	Y W Y F D L	0.14
Jh3	D A F D V	0.29
Jh4	Y F D Y	−0.11
Jh5	N W F D S	−0.23
Jh6	Y Y Y Y Y G M D V	0.01

B

First Trimester — Jh1 Jh2 Jh3 Jh4 Jh5 Jh6
Second Trimester — Jh1 Jh2 Jh3 Jh4 Jh5 Jh6
Adult — Jh1 Jh2 Jh3 Jh4 Jh5 Jh6

Figure 6. (A) Germline encoded amino acid sequence and average hydropathicity of the mouse and human Jh segments (only the HCDR3 part of the J's is shown). Tyrosine residues forming clusters in the N terminus are underlined. (B) Jh utilization (in percent) in human ontogeny. 37 first trimester fetal liver, 117 second trimester fetal liver [21] and bone marrow and 99 adult blood [24] VDJCμ + transcripts were analyzed and the percentage of the transcripts utilizing each J segment is shown.

In the fetal and neonatal mouse where N addition is absent, the range of HCDR3 hydropathicity is entirely dependent on germline sequence and reading frame preference. Under these conditions, the preference for rearrangement at sites of sequence identity between D and J virtually ensures use of RF1 alone, thus the average hydropathicity is similar to that in the germline D segments in RF1, i.e., slightly hydrophilic and enriched for Tyr, Ser and Gly (Figure 7). In the adult, the average hydropathicity appears to shift further towards the neutral range in spite of the presence of N nucleotides, which would be expected to reduce the contribution of preferential D–J rearrangement sites as well as adding random nucleotides potentially encoding either charged or hydro-phobic sequence [21]. However, in spite of N addition, the preference for Tyr, Ser, and Gly continues, suggesting that receptor-influenced selection may also play a role.

In the human, N region addition can be found as early as eight weeks gesta-tion, and there is no evidence of preferential rearrangement to RF1 even in the absence of N nucleotides, perhaps because the 3' sequence of most DH's is not as similar to the 5' sequence of JH as is the case in mouse. N addition appears to be more extensive in human, generating more random sequence. The extensive

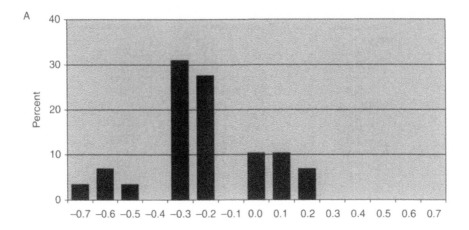

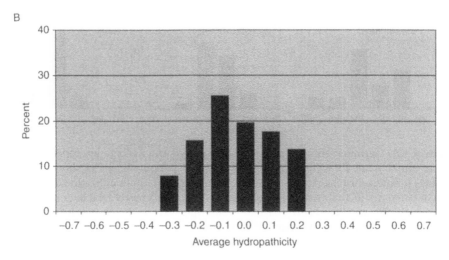

Figure 7. Comparison of the average hydropathicity of HCDR3 intervals in the mouse (from [28]): (A). Productive sequences from mouse newborn liver RNA (B). Productive sequences from mouse adult spleen RNA.

use of N addition and the absence of a bias for RF1 rearrangement in those sequences that lack N nucleotides might be predicted to allow greater variation in both RF usage and HCDR3 sequence composition and thus a greater range of hydropathicity in the HCDR3 interval. However, this does not occur. An evaluation of HCDR3 hydropathicity in DJ joins from fetal liver demonstrates the expected enhanced range of germline-based hydropathicity, due to more frequent use of alternative reading frames (Figure 8) [21]. However, few VDJ sequences contain the charged or hydrophobic HCDR3 sequences that would be expected from the hydropathicity of the DJ repertoire [21]. This adjustment in hydropathicity in part reflects exonucleolytic nibbling of the 5′ terminal nucleotides of the DH gene segments, limiting germline contribution of hydrophobic or charged amino acids. The extensive use of N addition between D and J also appears to allow a return to the neutral range [21, 34]. This

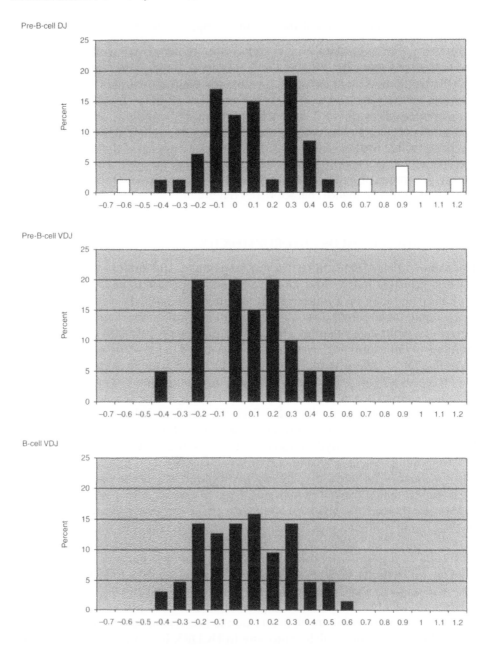

Figure 8. Adjustment of the hydropathicity of the human repertoire during B-cell development. Average HCDR3 hydropathicity of DJ and VDJ transcripts from pre-B and B-cells from second trimester fetal liver [21]. The highly charged and hydrophobic sequences seen only in DJ joins are represented in white.

modulation of hydropathicity as a consequence of germline nucleotide loss and the insertion of non-germline encoded sequence leaves open the possibility that receptor-based selection may play a significant role in restricting the use of hydrophobic or charged HCDR3 sequence.

The Mechanisms may Vary, but the End Result Appears to be the Same

In summary, the mechanisms used to prejudice or influence hydropathicity in mouse and human may vary, but the end result appears to be the same – generation of an HCDR3 repertoire that is restricted towards the neutral, hydrophilic range and is enriched for tyrosine, serine and glycine residues. In both species, the germline sequence prejudices the HCDR3 repertoire towards these three amino acids and against use of highly charged or hydrophobic amino acids (Figures 4 and 5). The mechanisms that further contribute to this preference appear to differ between both species and within a species and between the fetus and the adult. However, the outcome is generation of mouse and human antibody repertoires that share a surprising number of similar sequence characteristics (Figure 3).

III. EVOLUTION OF HCDR3 HYDROPATHICITY

The pattern of constraints in HCDR3 hydropathicity and amino acid composition that characterizes human and mouse antibodies appears to have arisen early in evolution, and may be a fundamental feature of an antibody repertoire. Various species may preferentially use alternative diversification mechanisms (e.g., gene conversion in the case of rabbit, chicken and pig), or present with a very different germline organization (e.g., *Heterodontus*) (reviewed in [35–37]). Nevertheless, the germ-line DH segments in all these species have the same general characteristics that were described in an earlier section for mouse and human (Figure 9). Germline segregation of hydropathicity by reading frame is a common feature. Preservation of hydropathicity is a reflection of amino acid preference, with RF1 in virtually all of these species enriched for glycine, tyrosine and serine; RF2 containing a high degree of hydrophobic amino acids, mainly valine and alanine; and RF3 containing Stop codons and enriched for leucine.

In functional VDJ joins, the slightly hydrophilic RF1 is the preferred reading frame in virtually all jawed vertebrates. Even in species with a very low number of D segments, such as catfish (3) and swine (2), where over-representation of one reading frame would be expected to further limit diversity, RF1 is utilized in more than 60% of cDNA sequences [38, 39]. This preference appears to be established very early in a number of species, as well as mice and humans (see above). In chicken, for example, 50% of embryonic DJ sequences are in RF1, and more than 90% of embryonic VDJs in the bursa are in-frame and in RF1 [40].

The amino acid composition of JH gene segments also appears to be conserved across evolution (refer Figure 9). In addition to preserving a preference for neutral, hydrophilic 5' termini, which contribute to HCDR3, in most species at least one JH gene segment begins with a cluster of tyrosine residues.

A preference for use of Tyr and Gly continues in the HCDR3 sequences of expressed VDJ structures. This was clearly documented by Golub *et al.* [41] in their analysis of amino acid utilization in the HCDR3 of four divergent species, (trout, axolotl, *Xenopus*, and mouse) (Figure 10). In all four species, Tyr and Gly account for at least 40% of the amino acids in HCDR3, including 54% of the amino acids in axolotl HCDR3 [41].

Axolotl appears to present an exception that emphasizes the rule. Although the germ-line sequences of the D segments are not known, 4 DH like elements have

Species	D	RF1	HP	RF2	HP	RF3	HP
Human	D6-13	GYSSSWY	-0.14	GIAAAG	+0.68	V*QQLV	+0.52
Mouse	DFL16.1	YYYGSSY	-0.18	FITTVVA	+0.95	LLLR**L	+0.86
Pig	DHB	DYSGCYSGY	-0.11	TIAVAIAV	+1.11	LRLL*RL	+0.50
Rabbit	D4	YYSSGWG	-0.12	VTIVVAGV	+1.10	LL**WLG	+0.82
Chicken	D6	GSGYCGSGAY	+0.12	VVVTVVVVL	+1.39	WLLW*WCL	+0.68
Xenopus	DH1	YASGYS	+0.01	TLAGT	+0.41	R*RVQ	-0.50
Axolotl	DH1	GGW	-0.03	GGL	+0.49	GA	+0.40
Catfish	D1	YSSWG	-0.12	VIAAGV	+1.08	L*QLG*	+0.46
Trout	DH4	NSGY	-0.34	IAGT	+0.61	*RVP	+0.09
Shark	DH1	YYSGY	-0.18	VLNWV	+0.69	GTTVG	+0.30

Species	J segment	HCDR3 portion	Hydropathicity
Human	JH6	YYYYYG M D V	+0.01
Mouse	JH4	YY A M D Y	-0.04
Pig	JH	L L C	+1.27
Rabbit	JH6	YY G M D L	+0.12
Chicken	JH	T E G S I D A	+0.30
Xenopus	JH5	YY A F D Y	+0.01
Axolotl	JH2	YYY F D Y	-0.16
Catfish	JH2	YY S Y F D Y	-0.15
Trout	JHB	YY F D Y	-0.14
Salmon	JH1-1	YY F D Y	-0.14

Figure 9. Comparison of germ-line heavy chain gene segments from various vertebrates. Representative D and J segments for each species are shown together with the calculated relative hydropathicity. The preferred reading frame of the D segment is bold. For the J segments sequences with clusters of tyrosines at the amino-terminus were selected, and the clustered Y residues are underlined. HP = hydropathicity.

D and J segment sequences from:
Human - [22, 55]
Mouse - [55]
Pig - [56, 39]
Rabbit - [57]
Chicken - [40]
Xenopus - [58, 64]
Axolotl - [59, 41]
Catfish - [38, 60]
Trout - [63, 62, 61]
Shark - [29]
Salomon - [55]

been identified from cDNA. They are very short and, unlike the other species, lack tyrosine, although they are enriched for glycine in all reading frames (Figure 9). However, axolotl JH segments are longer than those found in the other species, and their sequence is highly enriched for Tyr residues (Figure 10) [41]. Again, specific mechanisms often differ, but the end result remains the same.

The end result of immunoglobulin gene segment rearrangement and early B cell development in virtually all species examined to date is the generation of an HCDR3 repertoire where neutral or slightly charged amino acids are common, and charged or hydrophobic amino acids are rare. The range of hydropathicity in these various species is thus generally restricted (Figure 11). Generation of neutral or slightly hydrophilic HCDR3s appears to be a common feature in the active antibody repertoire that appeared early in evolution and has been preserved in spite of species-specific differences in diversification mechanisms.

POTENTIAL CONSEQUENCES OF A RESTRICTED HCDR3 REPERTOIRE FOR THE NORMAL, AND ABNORMAL, FUNCTION OF THE IMMUNE SYSTEM

It is a fundamental tenet of molecular biology that conservation of sequence across evolution marks selection for function. Why then might the sequence composition and hydropathicity of diversity (DH) and joining (JH) gene segments be preserved in the germline; and why, in spite of the opportunity given by N addition for further diversification, does the hydropathicity of HCDR3 remain constrained in the final repertoire?

Use of Charged or Hydrophobic HCDR3 Intervals could be Generally Deleterious

On the one hand, use of charged or hydrophobic amino acids could be deleterious to the normal function of the immune response. First, use of hydrophobic or charged amino acids may be more likely to generate HCDR3 intervals that preclude normal H chain function. Difficulties could arise in the formation of a stable H chain, a functional pre-B cell receptor, or a functional IgM molecule and thus block B cell development [42].

A second possibility is that use of alternative reading frames and the amino acids they encode is discouraged as a result of the antigen binding properties of

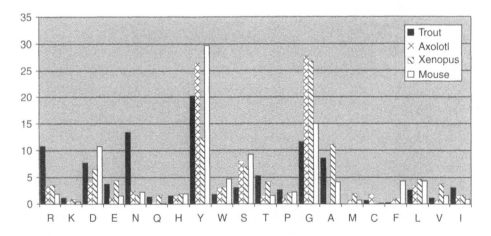

Figure 10. Percentages of amino acids in HCDR3 of four species as documented by Golub *et al.* [41]

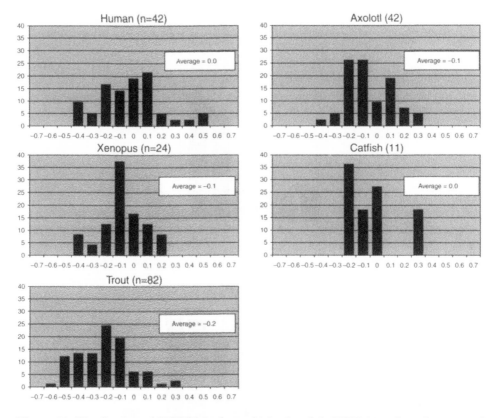

Figure 11. Distribution of HCDR3 hydropathicity in adult V(D)J joins from human and several lower vertebrates. N – number of sequences analyzed.
The sequences were taken from the following references:

Human -   [23]
Axolotl - [41]
Xenopus - [64]
Trout -   [62]
Catfish - [38]

the mature antibody. For example, use of alternative reading frames could yield stable but non-protective antibodies to specific antigens. Hydrophobic HCDR3 domains might be less likely to bind soluble antigens, such as polysaccharides or the surface of a virus, a parasite, or a toxin. Water molecules play an important role in bridging antigen and antibody [43]. A hydrophilic HCDR3 could facilitate the bridging action of water. Hydrophobic HCDR3 intervals might be discouraged because they would be less likely to create such bridges, generating antibodies that would be unable to protect against certain antigens. Alternatively, antibodies using RF2 and generating hydrophobic sequence might bind the wrong type of antigens. Antibody repertoires generated *in vitro* that contain hydrophobic HCDR3 intervals can also yield a high frequency of self-reactive antibodies, having a tendency to indiscriminately bind denatured protein (A. Plueckthun, personal communication).

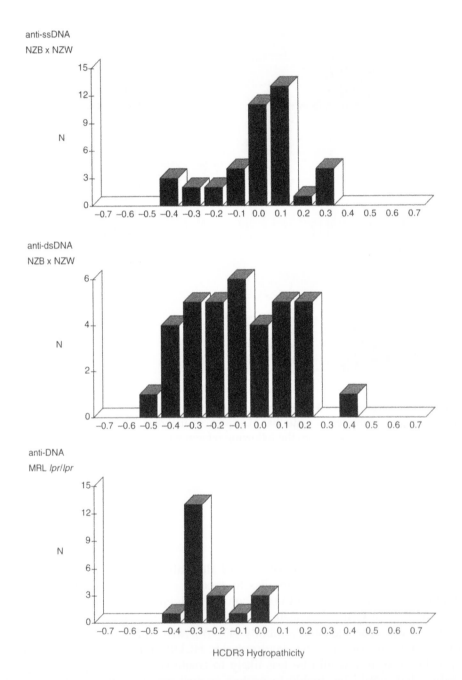

Figure 12. Hydropathicity of HCDR3 among anti-DNA antibodies. Shown are average hydropathicity values for HCDR3 intervals from a compilation of anti-DNA sequences from NZB × NZW mice [45] distributed into antibodies that recognize anti-single stranded DNA (top) and anti-double stranded DNA (middle). Shown at the bottom are average hydropathicity values for HCDR3 intervals from anti-DNA antibodies cloned from MRL *lpr/lpr* mice [44].

Charged HCDR3 domains might also be more likely to bind antigen indiscriminately, through salt bridges, or bind to self-antigen too well. A characteristic feature of anti-DNA antibodies, and especially anti-double stranded DNA antibodies, is the presence of arginine residues in the hypervariable domains, and especially HCDR3. These residues result in the generation of charged HCDR3 domains, particularly among anti-dsDNA antibodies (Figure 12) [45, 44]. This observation led Weigert and colleagues to suggest that reading frame preference for RF1 primarily serves to limit charge, thus reducing the likelihood of generating pathogenic autoantibodies [44].

Given evolutionary reluctance to use charged amino acids in D_H and J_H gene segments, in the mouse the presence of charged amino acids in HCDR3 are typically the product of N addition (refer Figure 5). This fact may help interpret the results of an analysis of anti-DNA antibodies in an autoimmune prone strain of mice (NZB × NZW) that were bred to contain a null mutant of TdT. In these mice VDJ joins lacked N addition and both anti-ss and anti-ds DNA antibodies were generated. However, many of these mice demonstrated no evidence of renal inflammation or other overt signs of renal disease [46]. Thus, the development of nephritis is not simply due to the production of anti-ds DNA antibodies, but to the production of the right, or wrong, types of anti-ds DNA antibodies. In these mice, pre-immune HCDR3 intervals with charged amino acids would be expected to be even more rare due to the absence of N addition.

The MRL-*lpr/lpr* [47] mouse serves as a classic model of systemic lupus erythematosus (SLE). This strain carries the *lpr* mutation, a loss-of-function allele of the *Fas* apoptosis gene (CD95), in addition to several other genetic defects. The general phenotype of the MRL-*lpr/lpr* mouse includes massive lymphadenopathy, hypergammaglobulinemia, glomerular nephritis, and high titers of autoantibodies to a variety of self-antigens, including chromatin, snRNP, and DNA [48, 49]. Recent studies have shown that the HCDR3 pre-immune repertoire of MRL-*lpr/lpr* mice, has an altered reading frame preference (only 9 of 19 VDJ sequences in RF1) [50], adding support to the view that alteration of HCDR3 hydropathicity may be deleterious to the organism by increasing the likelihood of generating pathogenic autoantibodies.

Use of Neutral, Hydrophilic HCDR3 Intervals could be Beneficial

A significant component of antibody in the blood of adults also belongs to the poorly understood category of "natural autoantibodies". These poly self-reactive antibodies, which are felt to be primarily the product of the B-1 B cell population, include much of the IgM anti-polysaccharide repertoire. This poly-reactive repertoire could thus be a throwback to a more primitive immune system that has been maintained across evolution in order to function as the first line of defense against infection, especially against encapsulated organisms, thus serving as an "evolutionary memory B cell" population. In the mouse, the neonatal antibody repertoires and the majority of the B-1 repertoires to be first described contain HCDR3 intervals that have few N additions and are thus highly enriched for hydrophilic, neutral amino acids derived from D_H sequence in RF1 [28, 32]. It is possible that the need to generate the "natural autoantibody" repertoire, which is over-represented among the B-1 subpopulation, has provided the evolutionary drive to preserve D_H sequence and generate hydrophilic HCDR3 domains.

A second possibility is that neutral hydrophilic sequences are more likely to encode protective antibodies against pathogens common to all vertebrate species. For example, in the BALB/c mouse, the T-independent antigen phosphoryl-choline (PC) [52] elicits a dominant idiotypic response, the T15 idiotype. Antibodies expressing the T15 idiotype provide protection from infection with *S. pneumoniae*, whereas mice that lack antibodies with this idiotype are susceptible and are more likely to perish after exposure to this encapsulated bacterium [53]. The T15 idiotype is germline encoded and thus is neutral, hydrophilic, and enriched for Gly, Tyr, and Ser residues.

SUMMARY

The conservation of HCDR3 sequence preference among vertebrates of widely divergent groups suggests evolutionary selection for function, but whether the conservation reflects positive or negative selection remains unclear. The proponents for positive selection would suggest that antibodies with neutral or slightly charged HCDR3s are preferred for proper binding of what are necessarily antigens with water-soluble surfaces. Proponents of negative selection would suggest that highly charged or hydrophobic sequences are deleterious. Potential deleterious effects include a reduced ability to form functional, stable proteins; an inability to bind necessary antigens; or a propensity to bind self-antigens. Distinguishing between these two possibilities will require a direct experimental test *in vivo*, through the generation of gene-targeted models with changed germline D segment repertoire (Ippolito *et al.* manuscript in preparation).

ACKNOWLEDGMENT

This work was supported by HD36292.

REFERENCES

1. Kirkham, P.M., and Schroeder, H.W., Jr. (1994). Antibody structure and the evolution of immunoglobulin V gene segments. *Semin. Immunol.* **6**, 347–360.
2. Kabat, E.A., Wu, T.T., Perry, H.M., Gottesman, K.S., and Foeller, C. (1991). Sequences of proteins of immunological interest. (Bethesda, Maryland: U.S. Department of Health and Human Services), pp. 1–2387.
3. Leder, P. (1982). The genetics of antibody diversity. *Scientific American* **246**(5), 102–115.
4. Tonegawa, S. (1983). Somatic generation of antibody diversity. *Nature* **302**, 575–581.
5. Honjo, T. (1983). Immunoglobulin genes. *Ann. Rev. Immunol.* **1**, 499–528.
6. Okada, A. and Alt, F.W. (1995). The variable region gene assembly mechanism. In Immunoglobulin Genes, T. Honjo and F.W. Alt, eds. (Academic Press), pp. 205–234.
7. Alt, F.W., Oltz, E.M., Young, F., Gorman, J., Taccioli, G., and Chen, J. (1992). VDJ recombination. [Review] [88 refs]. *Immunol. Today* **13**, 306–314.
8. Grawunder, U., West, R.B., and Lieber, M.R. (1998). Antigen receptor gene rearrangement [see comments]. [Review] [69 refs]. *Curr. Opin. Immunol.* **10**, 172–180.
9. Kehoe, J.M. and Capra, J.D. (1974). Phylogenetic aspects of immunoglobulin variable region diversity. *Contemp. Top. Mol. Immunol.* **3**, 143–159.

10. Shiokawa, S., Mortari, F., Lima, J.O., Nunez, C., Bertrand, F.E., III, Kirkham, P.M., Zhu, S., Dasanayake, A.P., and Schroeder, H.W., Jr. (1999). IgM heavy chain complementarity-determining region 3 diversity is constrained by genetic and somatic mechanisms until two months after birth. *J. Immunol.* **162**, 6060–6070.

11. Wu, T.T., Johnson, G., and Kabat, E.A. (1993). Length distribution of CDRH3 in antibodies. *Prot. Struct. Func. Genet.* **16**, 1–7.

12. Rock, E.P., Sibbald, P.R., Davis, M.M., and Chien, Y.H. (1994). CDR3 length in antigen-specific immune receptors. *J. Exp. Med.* **179**, 323–328.

13. Silverstein, A.M. (1977). Ontogeny of the Immune Response: A Perspective. In Development of Host Defense, M.D.Cooper, ed. (New York: Raven Press), pp. 1–10.

14. Schroeder, H.W., Jr. and Perlmutter, R.M. (1993). Development of the human antibody repertoire. S.Gupta and C.Griscelli, eds. (Chichester: New Concepts in Immunodeficiency Diseases), pp. 1–20.

15. Schroeder, H.W., Jr., Mortari, F., Shiokawa, S., Kirkham, P.M., Elgavish, R.A., and Bertrand, F.E.I. (1995). Developmental regulation of the human antibody repertoire. *Ann. N. Y. Acad. Sci.* **764**, 242–260.

16. Paton, J.C., Toogood, I.R., Cockington, R.A., and Hansman, D.J. (1986). Antibody response to pneumococcal vaccine in children aged 5 to 15 years. *Am. J. Dis. Child.* **140**, 135–138.

17. Stein, K.E. (1992). Thymus-independent and thymus-dependent responses to polysaccharide antigens. *J. Inf. Dis.* **165**, S49–S52.

18. Tuaillon, N. and Capra, J.D. (2000). Evidence that terminal deoxynucleotidyltransferase expression plays a role in Ig heavy chain gene segment utilization. *J. Immunol.* **164**, 6387–6397.

19. Gauss, G.H., and Lieber, M.R. (1996). Mechanistic constraints on diversity in human V(D)J recombination. *Mol. Cell Biol.* **16**, 258–269.

20. Marshall, A.J., Doyen, N., Bentolila, L.A., Paige, C.J., and Wu, G.E. (1998). Terminal deoxynucleotidyl transferase expression during neonatal life alters D(H) reading frame usage and Ig-receptor-dependent selection of V regions. *J. Immunol.* **161**, 6657–6663.

21. Schroeder, H.W., Jr., Ippolito, G.C., and Shiokawa, S. (1998). Regulation of the antibody repertoire through control of HCDR3 diversity. *Vaccine* **16**, 1383–1390.

22. Corbett, S.J., Tomlinson, I.M., Sonnhammer, E.L.L., Buck, D., and Winter, G. (1997). Sequence of the human immunoglobulin diversity (D) segment locus: a systematic analysis provides no evidence for the use of DIR segments, inverted D segments, "minor" D segments or D-D recombination. *J. Mol. Biol.* **270**, 587–597.

23. Raaphorst, F.M., Raman, C.S., Tami, J., Fischbach, M., and Sanz, I. (1997). Human Ig heavy chain CDR3 regions in adult bone marrow pre-B-cells display an adult phenotype of diversity: evidence for structural selection of DH amino acid sequences. *Int. Immunol.* **9**, 1503–1515.

24. Yamada, M., Wasserman, R., Reichard, B.A., Shane, S., Caton, A.J., and Rovera, G. (1991). Preferential utilization of specific immunoglobulin heavy chain diversity and joining segments in adult human peripheral blood B-lymphocytes. *J. Exp. Med.* **173**, 395–407.

25. Eisenberg, D. (1984). Three-dimensional structure of membrane and surface proteins. *Annu. Rev. Biochem.* **53**, 595–623.

26. Cornette, J.L., Cease, K.B., Margalit, H., Spouge, J.L., Berzofsky, J.A., and DeLisi, C. (1987). Hydrophobicity scales and computational techniques for detecting amphipathic structures in proteins. *J. Mol. Biol.* **195**, 659–685.

27. Kyte, J., and Doolittle, R.F. (1982). A simple method for displaying the hydropathic character of a protein. *J. Mol. Biol.* **157**, 105–132.

28. Feeney, A.J. (1990). Lack of N regions in fetal and neonatal mouse immunoglobulin V-D-J junctional sequences. *J. Exp. Med.* **172**, 1377–1390.

29. Hinds-Frey, K.R., Nishikata, H., Litman, R.T., and Litman, G.W. (1993). Somatic variation precedes extensive diversification of germline sequences and combinatorial joining in the evolution of immunoglobulin heavy chain diversity. *J. Exp. Med.* **178**, 815–824.

30. Davis, M.M., Lyons, D.S., Altman, J.D., McHeyzer-Williams, M., Hampl, J., Boniface, J.J., and Chien, Y. (1997). T cell receptor biochemistry, repertoire selection and general features of TCR and Ig structure. *Ciba Foundation Symposium* **204**, 94–100.

31. Sollbach, A.E., and Wu, G.E. (1995). Inversions produced during V(D)J rearrangement at IgH, the immunoglobulin heavy-chain locus. *Mol. Cell Biol.* **15**, 671–681.

32. Gu, H., Kitamura, D., and Rajewsky, K. (1991). B cell development regulated by gene rearrangement: arrest of maturation by membrane-bound Dmu protein and selection of DH element reading frames. *Cell* **65**, 47–54.

33. Nakamura, Y., Gojobori, T., and Ikemura, T. (2000). Codon usage tabulated from international DNA sequence databases: status for the year 2000. *Nucleic Acids Res.* **28**, 292.

34. Desiderio, S.V., Yancopoulos, G.D., Paskind, M., Thomas, E., Boss, M.A., Landau, N.R., Alt, F.W., and Baltimore, D. (1984). Insertion of N regions into heavy-chain gene is correlated with expression of terminal deoxytransferase in B-cells. *Nature* **311**, 752–755.

35. Knight, K.L., and Crane, M.A. (1995). Development of the antibody repertoire in rabbits. *Ann. N. Y. Acad. Sci.* **764**, 198–206.

36. Litman, G.W., Anderson, M.K., and Rast, J.P. (1999). Evolution of antigen binding receptors. *Annu. Rev. Immunol.* **17**, 109–147.

37. Weill, J.C., and Reynaud, C.A. (1995). Generation of diversity by post-rearrangement diversification mechanisms: the chicken and the sheep antibody repertoires. In Immunoglobulin Genes, T. Honjo and F.W. Alt, eds. Academic Press), pp. 267–288.

38. Hayman, J.R., and Lobb, C.J. (2000). Heavy chain diversity region segments of the channel catfish: structure, organization, expression and phylogenetic implications. *J. Immunol.* **164**, 1916–1924.

39. Sun, J., and Butler, J.E. (1996). Molecular characterization of VDJ transcripts from a newborn piglet. *Immunology* **88**, 331–339.

40. Reynaud, C.A., Anquez, V., and Weill, J.C. (1991). The chicken D locus and its contribution to the immunoglobulin heavy chain repertoire. *Eur. J. Immunol.* **21**, 2661–2670.

41. Golub, R., Fellah, J.S., and Charlemagne, J. (1997). Structure and diversity of the heavy chain VDJ junctions in the developing Mexican axolotl. *Immunogenetics* **46**, 402–409.

42. Raaphorst, F.M., Raman, C.S., Nall, B.T., and Teale, J.M. (1997). Molecular mechanisms governing reading frame choice of immunoglobulin diversity genes. *Immunol. Today* **18**, 37–43.

43. Mariuzza, R.A., and Poljak, R.J. (1993). The basics of binding: mechanisms of antigen recognition and mimicry by antibodies. *Curr. Opin. Immunol.* **5**, 50–55.

44. Shlomchik, M.J., Mascelli, M.A., Shan, H., Radic, M.Z., Pisetsky, D.S., Marshak-Rothstein, A., and Weigert, M.G. (1990). Anti-DNA antibodies from autoimmune mice arise by clonal expansion and somatic mutation. *J. Exp. Med.* **171**, 265–297.

45. Krishnan, M.R., Jou, N.T., and Marion, T.N. (1996). Correlation between the amino acid position of arginine in VH- CDR3 and specificity for native DNA among autoimmune antibodies. *J. Immunol.* **157**, 2430–2439.

46. Conde, C., Weller, S., Gilfillan, S., Marcellin, L., Martin, T., and Pasquali, J.L. (1998). Terminal deoxynucleotidyl transferase deficiency reduces the incidence of autoimmune nephritis in (New Zealand Black × New Zealand White) F1 mice. *J. Immunol.* **161**, 7023–7030.

47. Murphy, E.D., and Roths, J.B. (1999). In Topics in Hematology: Proceedings of the 16th International Congress in Hematology, S. Seno, F. Takaku, and S. Irino, eds. (Amsterdam: Excerpta Medica), pp. 69–72.

48. Theofilopoulos, A.N., and Dixon, F.J. (1985). Murine models of systemic lupus erythematosus. *Adv. Immunol.* **37**, 269–390.

49. Cohen, P.L., and Eisenberg, R.A. (1992). The lpr and gld genes in systemic autoimmunity: life and death in the Fas lane. *Immunol. Today* **13**, 427–428.
50. Alarcon-Riquelme, M.E., and Fernandez, C. (1995). CDR3 regions in the preimmune VH B cell repertoire of lpr mice. *Clin. Exp. Immunol.* **101**, 73–77.
51. Gu, H., Forster, I., and Rajewsky, K. (1990). Sequence homologies, N sequence insertion and JH gene utilization in VH-D-JH joining: implications for the joining mechanism and the ontogenetic timing of Ly1 B cell and B-CLL progenitor generation. *EMBO J.* **9**, 2133–2140.
52. Lieberman, R., Potter, M., Mushinski, E.B., Humphrey, W., Jr., and Rudikoff, S. (1974). Genetics of a new immunoglobulin VH (T15 idiotype) marker in the mouse regulating natural antibody to phosphorylcholine. *J. Exp. Med.* **139**, 983.
53. Briles, D.E., Nahm, M., Schroer, K., Davie, J., Baker, P., Kearney, J.F., and Barletta, R. (1981). Antiphosphocholine antibodies found in normal mouse serum are protective against intravenous infection with type 3 streptococcus pneumoniae. *J. Exp. Med.* **153**, 694–705.
54. Ichihara, Y., Hayashida, H., Miyazawa, S., and Kurosawa, Y. (1989). Only DFL16, DSP2, and DQ52 gene families exist in mouse immunoglobulin heavy chain diversity gene loci, of which DFL16 and DSP2 originate from the same primordial DH gene. *Eur. J. Immunol.* **19**, 1849–1854.
55. Ruiz, M., Giudicelli, V., Ginestoux, C., Stoehr, P., Robinson, J., Bodmer, J., Marsh, S.G., Bontrop, R., Lemaitre, M., Lefranc, G., Chaume, D., and Lefranc, M.P. (2000). IMGT, the international ImMunoGeneTics database. *Nucleic Acids Res.* **28**, 219–221.
56. Butler, J.E., Sun, J., and Navarro, P. (1996). The swine Ig heavy chain locus has a single JH and no identifiable IgD. *Int. Immunol.* **8**, 1897–1904.
57. Friedman, M.L., Tunyaplin, C., Zhai, S.K., and Knight, K.L. (1994). Neonatal VH, D, and JH gene usage in rabbit B lineage cells. *J. Immunol.* **152**, 632–641.
58. Mussmann, R., Courtet, M., and Du, P.L. (1998). Development of the early B cell population in Xenopus. *Eur. J. Immunol.* **28**, 2947–2959.
59. Fellah, J.S., Jacques, C., and Charlemagne, J. (1994). Characterization of immunoglobulin heavy chain variable regions in the Mexican axolotl. *Immunogenetics* **39**, 201–206.
60. Hayman, J.R., Ghaffari, S.H., and Lobb, C.J. (1993). Heavy chain joining region segments of the channel catfish. Genomic organization and phylogenetic implications. *J. Immunol.* **151**, 3587–3596.
61. Roman, T., Andersson, E., Bengten, E., Hansen, J., Kaattari, S., Pilstrom, L., Charlemagne, J., and Matsunaga, T. (1996). Unified nomenclature of Ig VH genes in rainbow trout (Oncorhynchus mykiss): definition of eleven VH families. *Immunogenetics* **43**, 325–326.
62. Roman, T., De Guerra, A., and Charlemagne, J. (1995). Evolution of specific antigen recognition: size reduction and restricted length distribution of the CDRH3 regions in the rainbow trout. *Eur. J. Immunol.* **25**, 269–273.
63. Roman, T., and Charlemagne, J. (1994). The immunoglobulin repertoire of the rainbow trout (Oncorhynchus mykiss): definition of nine Igh-V families. *Immunogenetics* **40**, 210–216.
64. Schwager, J., Burckert, N., Courtet, M., and Du, P.L. (1991). The ontogeny of diversification at the immunoglobulin heavy chain locus in Xenopus. *EMBO J.* **10**, 2461–2470.

Chapter

FOUR

Molecular Aspects of Anti-Polysaccharide Antibody Responses

Kurt Brorson, Pablo Garcia-Ojeda, and Kathryn E. Stein

Division of Monoclonal Antibodies, Center for Biologics Evaluation and Research, Food and Drug Administration, 29 Lincoln Drive, Bethesda MD 20892–4555, USA

I. INTRODUCTION

Scope of Review

Polysaccharides (PS) are a diverse set of molecules present in all living cells, serving a myriad of functions. PS range from simple polymers of one type of sugar to complex structures of multiple sugars and linkages. Additional complexity in carbohydrate structure arises from glycosylation of proteins and lipids with complex oligosaccharides. In bacteria, PS structures are found in cell walls as long repeating chains, on many endotoxins and as capsules. The capsules on human pathogens act as virulence factors and protect the organism from non-specific host defense mechanisms. Antibody (Ab) responses against PS are qualitatively different than immune responses to other antigens (e.g., proteins) (1). PS contain repetitive sugar epitopes which influence the mechanism of immune activation and the nature of the resulting antibodies.

Research over several decades on anti-PS immune responses has greatly impacted medicine and public health. Specific antibody responses against the capsular PS of *Haemophilus influenzae*, *Neisseria meningitidis* and *Streptococcus pneumoniae* and other encapsulated bacteria are critical for host protection against invasive disease, but are sub-optimal in certain at-risk populations, e.g., infants. A major effort in investigating the immunology of bacterial capsular PS has lead recently to the introduction of improved PS vaccines through the use of PS–protein conjugates. These conjugate vaccines elicit more robust anti-capsular antibody responses and provide better protection to susceptible populations. In the field of cancer, abnormal glycosylation patterns of cell surface glycoproteins or glycolipids have been studied as markers for transformation. Antibodies specific for these carbohydrate tumor antigens are being developed as less toxic alternatives to conventional chemotherapy. Because of their roles in protective immunity against encapsulated bacteria and their potential therapeutic uses for passive protection and as anti-tumor agents, anti-PS antibodies have become increasingly important to understand from the point of stimulating anti-PS responses as well as engineering antibodies to PS for high affinity. This review will discuss the immunology of responses to PS and the available data on the repertoire and structures of antibodies to a number of polysaccharide antigens.

Murine and human immunoglobulin variable regions have been classified into gene families based on hybridization experiments and amino acid sequence data (e.g., J558, J606, etc.; [2–5]). Recent genomic sequencing efforts have characterized each human V_H and mouse V_L gene, and a database of known mouse and human V region sequences has been compiled by the National Center for Biotechnology Information (NCBI/NIH; www.ncbi.nlm.nih.gov/igblast [6–14]). To maintain consistency of V gene terminology in this review, we have identified individual V genes (in parentheses) based on the NCBI database nomenclature (Table 1).

Nature of Anti-PS Responses

Anti-PS immune responses are unique in the nature of the B-cell activation signal. Unlike thymus-dependent (TD) antigens (e.g., proteins), T-cells are not required for immune activation, although other cell types and cytokines may be involved (e.g., NK cells [15]). Because of the lack of T-cell involvement, anti-PS responses are termed thymus-independent (TI). TI antigens are further sub-classified as type 1 TI antigens (TI-1, e.g., endotoxins) and type 2 TI antigens (TI-2, e.g., capsular PS) based on their ability to elicit antibody responses from *xid* immunodeficient mice (TI-1) and their inability to stimulate antibody responses in neonates (TI-2) (1). The unique characteristics of TI-2 responses *in vivo* are believed to reflect a distinct B-cell signaling mechanism. Unlike other antigens, TI-2 antigens possess repeating saccharide epitopes which are believed to directly activate B-Cells by cross-linking surface Ig receptors.

Antibodies elicited by TI-2 immune activation are qualitatively different from antibodies to TD antigens. Immunization with simple PS elicit homogenous, usually germline, antibody responses using one or a few V_H:V_L pairs. Ab responses to more complex capsular PS are oligoclonal, with several V_H:V_L pairs represented in the antibody population and clonotypes are often limited within individuals. Certain V region genes appear to be over-represented among anti-PS Abs (e.g., V_HGal55.1). It is tempting to speculate that the smaller number of antigenic epitopes on PS with repeating antigenic determinants selects for more limited numbers of V_H:V_L pairs. Perhaps the limited V gene usage reflects a preference for certain complementarity determining region (CDR) topologies or residues [16]. However, this hypothesis does not fully explain the population level diversity of anti-capsular PS responses. Further, more broad V region usage can be generated using TD protein-conjugate forms of PS antigens.

It has been repeatedly observed that anti-PS antibodies have low avidity ($\sim 10^4$–10^6 M^{-1}) for antigen, although higher avidity antibodies can be elicited by TD PS–protein conjugates or repeated immunizations with pure PS [17]. Antigen binding involves multiple non-covalent interactions between atoms in the antigen and the CDR surface [18]. The residues in the CDR regions form loops, H1–3 in the heavy chain and L1–L3 in the light chain, between the strands of the β-pleated sheet of the immunoglobulin domain. Presumably, immunization with conjugates elicits somatic mutation increasing the number and quality of contacts between loop residues and PS. Recent three-dimensional (3-D) structural analysis of anti-PS antibodies, including some in contact with antigen, has suggested that aromatic residues on the CDR surface play an important role in binding to neutral PS antigens [19, 20]. In contrast, basic residues are involved with binding to negatively charged PS [21, 22]. An important structural consideration for PS binding is the surface topography of the CDR regions (e.g., "groove-type" vs. "cavity-type"; [23]).

Anti-PS antibodies tend to be IgM isotype and restricted IgG and IgA isotypes (e.g., IgG3 in mice, [24]; IgG2 in humans [25]; IgA in myeloma proteins, [26]). Ab isotype has been demonstrated to impact host protection against PS encapsulated pathogens. For example, μ-isotype Abs have been reported to be more effective in protection against PS-encapsulated pathogens (e.g., group B *Streptococcus*, *E. coli* K1) than γ-isotype Abs [27]. In another case, switching an anti-capsular PS antibody from γ3 to γ1 enhanced protection of mice against *Cryptococcus neoformans* [28]. It could be speculated that the lack of T-cell involvement in PS responses leads to the limited cytokine driven class switching to other IgG subclasses (e.g., IgG1, IgG2a, IgG2b).

Secondary responses to PS are limited in magnitude relative to those against proteins, although the formation of germinal centers in response to immunization with dextran has been described [29]. Somatic mutations in anti-PS Abs in response to TI-2 antigens are not common, although they are more extensive in Abs elicited by repeat immunization with pure PS [17] or by protein–PS conjugates [30]. Somatic mutations in anti-carbohydrate Abs are particularly evident in auto-antigen binding paraproteins, where the immunologic process behind their generation is poorly understood and are likely to be complex [31, 32].

The ability to mount TI-2 responses develops late in ontogeny in most cases (8–12 weeks of age in mice and 18–24 months in humans). The waning of maternal antibodies coupled with the inability of infants and young children to respond to PS antigens correlates with a high incidence of invasive disease, such as meningitis, caused by encapsulated pathogens. To overcome this problem, TD conjugate vaccines for *H. influenzae* type B (Hib) were introduced in the early 1990's and have nearly eliminated invasive *Haemophilus* disease in susceptible populations [33, 34]. A multivalent conjugate vaccine for *S. pneumoniae* has recently been licensed by CBER/FDA, and others are currently under development. It is clear that the use of TD forms of PS vaccines which stimulate higher affinity antibody and memory responses are a major public health advance for infant protection against the most common forms of infant meningitis caused by *H. influenzae* and the common capsular types of *S. pneumoniae*.

Table 1. Variable Region Usage in Mouse and Human Anti-PS Ab Responses

PS type	PS antigen	Predominant V$_H$ family[a]	V$_H$ gene(s)[b]	Predominant V$_L$ family[a]	V$_L$ gene(s)[b]	Minor V$_H$/V$_L$ genes and pairs[c]	References
Environmental PS (murine)	BL (In⁻)[d]	X24	Gal55.1	κ10	ce9	X24:κ4; J558:κ4	[42]
		V-GAM		λ1	L1	J558:λ; 36–09:λ; 36–60:κ; J606:λ	[17, 42, 43]
	BL (In⁺)[d]	J606	22.1	κ11	if11	J559:κ20; J558:κ11	[17, 43]
	Galactan	X24	Gal55.1	κ4	kb4		[44,76]
	Dextran B512F (pure PS)	J558	45.21.1, 132.26, 102	κ4	kk4	J606; Q52	[45]
	Dextran B512F (adjuvants)	J558	6, 23, 45.21.1, 132.26, 102	κ4	kk4, kn4	J558:κ1; J558:κ2; 36–60; X24:κ1; J606:κ4	[46, 48, 49]
	Dextran B1355S	J558	45.21.1	λ1	L1		[47, 82]
Capsular PS (murine)	MCPS[e]	J558	4 genes	κ		36–60; 3609; 7183; VGAM3–8; X24	[30, 151]
	Streptococcus group A	J606	22.1	κ24	he24, hf24	J606:κ2, λ	[155, 157]
	Cryptococcus serotype D	X24	Gal55.1	λ2	L2	7183:κ5.1; X24:λ1	[198]
	Cryptococcus serotype A[e]	7183	50.1	κ5.1	bb1	10:κ21; VGAM: κ4/5;11:κser	[199, 201]
Cell surface PS (murine)	Fucosyllactosamine	X24	Gal55.1	κ24	he24		[226]

	Gangliosides with NeuAcα(2→3) or (2→8)	J558					[230]
	Gangliosides with NeuAcα(2→6)	Q52					[230]
	Gangliosides with NeuAcα(2→9)	J606					[230]
	Galactosylgloboside	X24	Gal55.1	κOx-1 (κ4)	ai4		[231]
Capsular PS (human)	Hib CP[e]	Subgroup III	3-23, 3-15, 3-49	κII	A2	κI; κII; κIII; κIV; λI; λIII; λVII	[113–120, 123]
	S. pneumoniae 6F CP	Subgroup III					[186]
Cell surface (human)	Cold agglutinin i	Subgroup IV	4-34	κI	O2	κIII, λ	[235, 236]
	Cold agglutinin I	Subgroup IV	4-34	κIII	L2, A11		[235, 236, 245]

[a] Predominant V gene usage identified in reference or in re-analysis of publicly available sequence data (e.g., Genbank). For some PS systems discussed in this article, insufficient sequence data is available to identify predominant gene usage (e.g., MBPS, Streptococcus group B).

[b] Genes identified by Ig Blast (NCBI/NLM/NIH) using publicly available sequence data.

[c] Additional V genes or V_H:V_L pairs identified in reference or in re-analysis of publicly available sequence data.

[d] In[+] antibodies defined as reactive with β(2→1) levan (inulin).

[e] Includes Abs generated following immunization with PS-protein.

Further, these vaccines clearly demonstrate the protective role of anti-capsular antibodies.

II. ENVIRONMENTAL PS

Because of the ubiquitous presence of PS antigens in the environment, humans and mice develop "natural antibodies" to a variety of PS determinants. Exceptions are humans with Wiskott Aldrich syndrome who have antibody abnormalities and are at increased risk for diseases caused by *H. influenzae* and *S. pneumoniae* [35] and *xid* mice who fail to develop antibodies to PS [36]. Extensive research has been performed to examine antibody responses to environmental PS such as dextrans, galactans and levans. These PS are useful as model antigens for examining anti-PS immune responses because they are highly immunogenic TI-2 antigens yet simple in structure, eliciting antibodies against one or a few epitopes. They are polymers of a single or at most a few types of sugars, connected by a limited number of linkages and branching structures. Natural forms of these PS are by-products of microbial fermentation (e.g., levans and dextrans) or are present in tree exudate gums (e.g., galactans), allowing their isolation in more than sufficient quantities for immunological experimentation. Pure synthetic oligosaccharide counterparts of these PS can be synthesized for epitope mapping and attachment to protein carriers can convert them to TD antigens.

Mouse myeloma proteins, many of which are specific for environmental PS, were useful in early studies of anti-PS Ab biochemistry. A large fraction of myeloma proteins isolated from mouse tumors were identified as possessing specificity for dextrans, levans, or galactans. It was surmised that inbred mice develop natural anti-PS antibodies as they age because of constant environmental exposure (e.g., bacteria, food, bedding; [37, 38]). This notion is supported by the observation that mice housed under germ-free conditions and fed chemically defined ultrafiltered diets fail to produce normal levels of natural anti-levan or dextran antibodies [39, 40]. Amino acid sequencing of small collections of anti-dextran, levan or galactan myelomas revealed restricted usage of $V_H:V_L$ pairs, often with germline sequences. Myeloma proteins were almost universally found to possess modest affinity ($\sim 10^5$ M^{-1}) for PS antigen. PS epitope structures were identified (e.g., linear, internal epitopes vs. terminal sugar epitopes) and contact residues (e.g., Trp residues) were defined by fluorescence absorbence experiments [41]. Finally, their early availability has established myeloma proteins as references for subsequent studies and has provided names for variable region families (e.g., $V_H J606$, $V_H X24$, $V_H J558$), based on the plasmacytoma first used to define the V_H gene family.

Panels of hybridomas generated following PS immunization have proved to be another valuable tool to understand the genetics and fine specificity of anti-polysaccharide antibodies. With hybridomas, larger numbers of antibody secreting clones are available, and the immunization strategy can be controlled. As in the collections of myeloma proteins, IgM mAb and certain $V_H:V_L$ pairings predominate. However, because of panel size (up to 100 hybridomas) and variations in immunization method (e.g., different mouse strains, repeat immunizations, use of adjuvants), minor $V_H:V_L$ pairings have been isolated as well [42–49]. Presumed somatic mutations were identified in some mAbs, particularly those produced after secondary immunization. Mouse strain differences in $V_H:V_L$ usage and fine specificity were identified in several cases; some genetically mapping to Igh alleles, others to yet unidentified loci.

Levan

Levans are neutral polymers of fructose joined by either $\beta(2 \rightarrow 6)$ or $\beta(2 \rightarrow 1)$ linkages. Plant levans, made for energy storage, are linear polymers with either predominantly $\beta(2 \rightarrow 6)$ linkages (monocotyledons, e.g., rye grass) or predominantly $\beta(2 \rightarrow 1)$ linkages, also known as inulin (dicotyledons, e.g., Jerusalem artichokes; [50]). Bacterial levans (BL) are extra-cellular products of microbial fermentation by *Bacillus* and *Erwinia sp.* bacteria which synthesize levan from sucrose and secrete it [51]. BL is much larger ($M_r > 10^6$ Daltons) than plant levans, is readily soluble in water, and consists of a backbone of $\beta(2 \rightarrow 6)$ linked fructose with branches of $\beta(2 \rightarrow 1)$-linked fructose.

More than a dozen levan binding myeloma proteins have been isolated and characterized for fine specificity [52]. Two discrete fine specificities were identified among these levan-binding myeloma proteins; inulin reactive (e.g., J606, E109, A4, A47, U61, others) and inulin non-reactive (e.g., UPC10, A48). Affinity measurements of these proteins revealed that they have modest affinity for levan ($\sim 10^5 M^{-1}$, [53]), with maximal binding of oligosaccharides 3 and 4 sugars in length [53, 54]. Variable region sequencing of some of these myelomas revealed that V region usage differs with fine specificity. Inulin reactive antibodies (e.g., J606, U61, E109, A4 and A47) use one $V_H:V_L$ pair, V_HJ606:Vκ11 (V_H22.1:Vκif 11; [55, 56]) while inulin non-reactive antibodies (e.g., UPC10 and A48) use another, V_HX24:Vκ10 (V_HGal55.1:Vκ ce9; (57)). Interestingly, $\beta(2 \rightarrow 1)$ and $\beta(2 \rightarrow 6)$ levan are sufficiently similar, structurally, that J606 has a dual specificity in that it also binds pure $\beta(2 \rightarrow 6)$ levan purified from rye grass (GL, [58]). A model constructed of E109 provides a possible explanation of the cross-recognition [56]. E109, like the other V_HJ606:Vκ11 myelomas, has a uniquely short V_H CDR3 encoded H3 loop and is predicted to have a "cavity-like" binding site, able to accommodate both "bulky" $\beta(2 \rightarrow 1)$ and extended "ribbon-like" $\beta(2 \rightarrow 6)$ levans [59].

Data from panels of $\beta(2 \rightarrow 6)$ levan specific hybridomas have upheld the correlation between V_HX24:Vκ10 pairing and $\beta(2 \rightarrow 6)$ fine specificity, but have also identified other $\beta(2 \rightarrow 6)$ levan binding pairings [42]. Seven of nine hybridomas from BL immunized 129/sv mice were V_HX24:Vκ10, with two others being V_HX24:Vκ 4 and V_HJ558:Vκ4. Usage of V_HX24:Vκ10 and V_HX24:Vκ 4 pairs was also found among hybridomas produced by mixed immunization of BALB/c mice with anti-idiotype antibodies and BL [60]. The mixed immunization panel was very diverse in fine specificity in that despite being V_HX24:Vκ10, the Abs possessed several combinations of reactivities as evaluated with $\beta(2 \rightarrow 6)$ grass levan (GL), BL and inulin [61]. For example, UPC10, specific for $\beta(2 \rightarrow 6)$ levan bound GL and BL, but not inulin. MAb 2-1-3 binds all three in a manner similar to J606. MAb 3-27-6 bound GL, but not the other forms, while mAb 2-13-10 bound only BL. BL immunized κ-chain deficient 129 mice also produce anti-$\beta(2 \rightarrow 6)$ levan binding λ-chain mAbs with pairing not found in the 129/sv panel [42]. The majority (9/12) of the mAbs in this panel were V_HGAM:V$_\lambda$1 antibodies, while the remainder used V_HJ558 and V_H36–09 in conjunction with λ-light chains. Thus, in the absence of

K-light chains, the dominant $V_H X24:V\kappa10$ antibody response to $\beta(2 \rightarrow 6)$ levan can be replaced by $V_H GAM:V_\lambda 1$ antibodies.

Larger panels of hybridomas (~50 each) from BL immunized BALB/C and CBA/Ca mice were characterized by another lab [17, 43]. Both strains produced mostly IgM antibodies. Heterogeneity was evident in fine specificity (e.g., inulin reactive vs. inulin non-reactive), and $V_H:V_L$ pair usage, but a pattern of strain difference was apparent. Both panels contained inulin non-reactive, $V_H X24:V\kappa10$ and $V_H GAM:V_\lambda 1$ antibodies similar to those detected in the 129/sv and K-chain deficient panels. The majority of mAbs in the BALB/c panel were similar to the J606 myeloma in that they were mostly germline $V_H J606:V\kappa11$ and inulin reactive. In contrast, the CBA/Ca panel did not contain $V_H J606:V\kappa11$ antibodies, instead they used other pairings not found in the BALB/c panel. These included inulin non-reactive $V_H 36$–$60:V\kappa$ and $V_H J606:V_\lambda$ antibodies and inulin reactive $V_H J558:V\kappa$ ($V_H 23:V\kappa bt20$) and $V_H J558:V\kappa11$ ($V_H 23:V\kappa if11$) Abs. The fine specificity of the $V_H J606:V_\lambda$ antibodies appear to similar to mAb 2-13-10 in that it binds BL but not GL or inulin, possibly because the two mAbs recognize a $\beta(2 \rightarrow 1)$–$\beta(2 \rightarrow 6)$ combination epitope [62].

Sequence analysis of the IgM BALB/c $V_H J606:V\kappa11$ hybridomas revealed apparent CDR somatic mutations which correlated with high avidity for inulin: N53H in V_H; N53I and S30N in Vκ, particularly in mAbs generated after two BL immunizations [17]. These same substitutions are found in the myeloma proteins (e.g., E109, U61, A4, A47; [55, 56]), arguing that the process of affinity maturation consistently selects for a small set of mutants that contribute to high avidity. Site directed mutagenesis studies demonstrated that these changes caused marked increases in inulin avidity (between 9- and 46-fold), which nearly accounted for the avidity of the highest avidity mAb in the panel (62). The mutations implicated in inulin avidity changes appear to reside at distant locations of the CDR surface (Figure 1), arguing that a large proportion of the CDR surface participates in inulin binding. Earlier studies of fluorescence changes during levan:E109 binding, argued that Trp residues (probably $33V_H$ or $37V_H$) are involved with binding to this neutral PS [53]. This observation together with evidence that the addition of an aromatic residue (N53H in V_H) increases Ab avidity 9-fold, supports the hypothesis that aromatic CDR residues appear to be critical for interaction with this neutral PS. Preliminary observations that changing $V_H 53$ to other aromatic residues such as Tyr or Trp also increases avidity provide support for this hypothesis [63]. In contrast, these same substitutions do not impact avidity for BL or GL, arguing that although these mAbs have a dual specificity, $V_H 53$ and V$\kappa 53$ are important for binding $\beta(2 \rightarrow 1)$ levan only.

The same series of experiments demonstrated that exchanging allele-specific $V_H J606$ residues or the H3 loop between the $V_H J606:V\kappa11$ BALB/c and the $V_H J606:V_\lambda$ CBA/Ca mAb resulted in either a fine specificity shift away from inulin (N53D in BALB/c mAb) or a total loss of BL binding (E50Q in BALB/c mAb, BALB/c H3 loop $\rightarrow$ CBA/Ca mAb), identifying residues critical for binding both forms of levan ($V_H 50$) or joining with V_λ to construct a CDR surface specific for the $\beta(2 \rightarrow 1)$-$\beta(2 \rightarrow 6)$ combination epitope. 3-D models suggested that $V_H 53$ and $V_L 53$, critical for binding to inulin only, reside near the edge of the CDR surface. In contrast, $V_H 50$ and the H3 loop, critical for binding other forms of levan, are in the $V_H:V_L$ junction area.

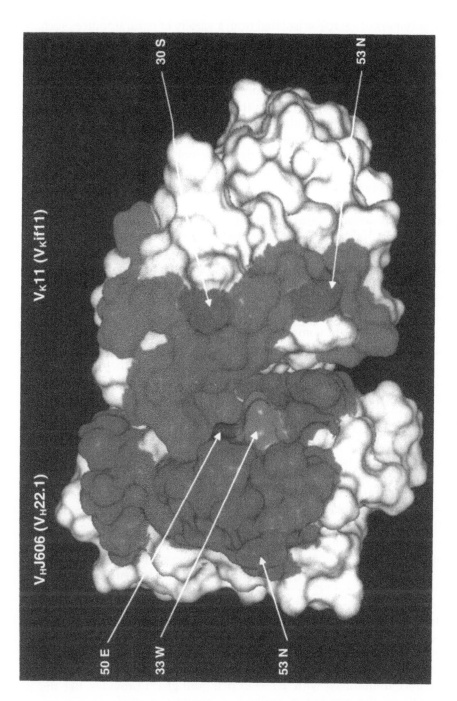

Figure 1. Molecular model of inulin binding mAb. Solvent accessible surface representation of the germline V_HJ606:$V_\kappa 11$ V region was constructed using the homology module of insight II 97.2 and the resolved PDB structures 1IAI (V_H), 1FVD (V_κ) and 1NSN (H3 loop; description of method is in [62]). The FR surface is colored white; the CDR surface green. Residues demonstrated by site directed mutagenesis studies to be involved in inulin binding are red [62], while Trp33H, suggested by fluorescence binding experiments to contact Ag, is colored ochre [53]. (See Color plate 2)

Galactan

Galactans are polymers of galactose isolated from a variety of natural sources such as plant tissues and exudates [64, 65], microbial sources [66] and animal mucosal tissues [67]. Plant galactans, sometimes referred to as arabinogalactans, are complexes consisting of an $\alpha(1 \to 3)$ or $\alpha(1 \to 6)$ linked galactan core and branch structures containing other sugars such as glucuronic acid, arabinose and rhamnose. Core linkage structures vary, depending on the natural source. For example, the galactan core of gum Ghatti (an exudate gum from *Anogeissus latifolia*) is mostly $\alpha(1 \to 6)$ linked while the galactan core of gum Arabic (an exudate gum from acacia trees) is mostly $\alpha(1 \to 3)$ linked [65, 68]. Synthetic polygalactans are available to determine antibody fine specificities in a manner more precise than possible with natural galactans [69, 70].

Six galactan binding myeloma proteins isolated to date (e.g., J539, T601, X24, X44, S10, and T191) demonstrate structural similarity in that they are all $V_H X24:V\kappa4$ ($V_H Gal55.1:V\kappa kb4$; [26, 44]). A limited degree of sequence heterogeneity is evident. Interestingly, many of these myelomas are of the IgA isotype. Of these myelomas, J539 has been most extensively characterized. J539 appears to possess an $\alpha(1 \to 6)$ galactan fine specificity, as binding to $\alpha(1 \to 6)$ and $\alpha(1 \to 3)$ containing larchwood arabinogalactan can be ablated by selective chemical degradation of the $\alpha(1 \to 6)$ linkages [71]. Early models of J539 predicted that it has a shallow antigen combining site, compatible with accommodation of a linear chain segment of galactan [72]. The observation that J539 effectively binds the nearly linear *Prototheca zopfii* $\alpha(1 \to 6)$ galactan corroborates the prediction that J539 binds the internal determinants of galactan that are abundant in this long-chain, non-branched form of galactan [71]. Additional binding studies with synthetic oligosaccharides also support this hypothesis [69, 70].

The early analysis of J539 provided some of the first insights into PS:Ig interactions. Galactan binding apparently involves aromatic residues on J539. Fluorescence absorbence changes occur upon Ag binding [73], and it was surmised that the fluorescence changes result from H bonds between PS and Trp residues on the CDR surface. The Trp fluorescence changes were also used to measure binding affinity; like other PS:Ig interactions, the affinity is modest ($10^5 \, M^{-1}$ [44]). Subsite mapping studies demonstrated optimal binding by galactan polymers of four sugars in length, each sugar in a separate CDR subsite denoted A-D (41). The structural resolution of the J539 Fab [74], in conjunction with the fluorescence absorbence observations, mapped the four subsites to a surface location formed by the L1, L3, H1 and H2 loops. The solvent accessible Trp residues presumed to contribute to antigen binding were identified as 91W in V_L and 33W in V_H. Using transferred nuclear Overhauser enhancement spectroscopy, it was demonstrated that the structure of galactan changes upon binding to the IgA myeloma X24 [75].

The galactan myelomas and a panel of five galactan binding mAbs generated from BALB/c mice immunized with $\alpha(1 \to 6)$ rich-gum ghatti provides, like the $V_H J606:V\kappa11$ pair in the anti-inulin antibodies, another example of extreme V region restriction in that all 11 use the $V_H X24:V\kappa4$ pair combination [76]. The largely IgM hybridoma antibodies displayed sequence variability, providing early evidence that somatic mutation is not always linked to class switching, as was observed recently for anti-inulin mAb [17].

Only by immunization with other plant galactans are anti-galactan antibodies produced that differ in fine specificity from the $V_H X24:V\kappa4$ myeloma proteins. Unfortunately, variable region sequence data from these mAbs are not available currently. One of these sets appears to preferentially bind a determinant composed of three $\alpha(1\rightarrow6)$ linked galactans and one arabinose [77]. The other set appears to be unique in binding gum Arabic, a complex exudate gum rich in $\alpha(1\rightarrow3)$ linked galactans [65, 78–80]. The gum Arabic binding mAb have a number of epitope fine specificities, and can be used to distinguish exudate gums [80].

Dextrans

Dextrans, exo-polysaccharide polymers of glucose produced by *Leuconostoc mesenteroides* bacteria, have been used as synthetic blood volume expanders [81]. Anti-dextran antibodies are clinically important because pre-existing anti-dextran antibodies, particularly antibodies reactive with non-$\alpha(1\rightarrow6)$ linkage dextran, correlate with anaphylactic reactions in patients given synthetic blood volume expanders. Dozens of strain specific dextrans exist, which differ in the relative proportion of $\alpha(1\rightarrow2)$, $\alpha(1\rightarrow3)$, $\alpha(1\rightarrow4)$, or $\alpha(1\rightarrow6)$ linkages. Two dextrans, B512F and B1355S, have been extensively characterized immunologically. B512F dextran contains mostly $\alpha(1\rightarrow6)$ linkages (90%) with 5% $\alpha(1\rightarrow3)$ branch linkages and 5% $(1\rightarrow)$ non-reducing end groups. B1355S dextran contains a high proportion of $\alpha(1\rightarrow3)$-$\alpha(1\rightarrow6)$ linear repeating linkages, with 10% $\alpha(1\rightarrow3)$ branch linkages and 10% $\alpha(1\rightarrow)$ non-reducing end groups. Because of their divergent linkage structures, antibody responses against both dextrans differ in $V_H:V_L$ usage. Synthetic polyglucans and nigerose, a poly-$\alpha(1\rightarrow3)$ glucose isolated from *Aspergillus niger*, are available for fine specificity analysis and to examine binding to pure $\alpha(1\rightarrow3)$ linkages.

Dextran binding myelomas display a broader range of fine specificities and $V_H:V_L$ pair combinations than either levan or galactan binding myelomas (e.g., J558, M104E, $V_H J558:V_\lambda1$; CAL20 TEPC1035, $V_H J558:\kappa$-isotype; W3129, $V_H X24:V\kappa1$; QUPC52, $V_H J558:V\kappa4$;[82–88]). Like the levan and galactan myelomas, the dextran binding proteins possess moderate affinity for antigen (10^5–10^6 M^{-1}; [89]). The dextran myelomas are specific either for linear $\alpha(1\rightarrow3)$–$\alpha(1\rightarrow6)$ repeating linkages present in B1355S dextran (e.g., J558, M104E), for $\alpha(1\rightarrow6)$ linkages as found in B512F dextran (e.g., W3129, QUPC52) or cross-reactive with B1355S dextran and dextran with $\alpha(1\rightarrow4)$–$\alpha(1\rightarrow6)$ repeating linkages (CAL20 TEPC1035). The $\alpha(1\rightarrow6)$ linkage specific Abs have been sub-categorized into those presumed to have "groove-type" CDR surfaces (reacting with internal parts of the $\alpha(1\rightarrow6)$ linked chain) and those presumed to have "cavity-type" CDR surfaces (reacting with terminal ends of the polymer). W3129 serves as a prototype "cavity type" myeloma while QUPC52 serves as a "groove-type" prototype [23]. Modeling studies of W3129 and a "groove-type" mAb 19.1.2, (encoded by $V_H6:V\kappa kk4$), predict that the relatively long V_L CDR1 encoded L1 domain and the V_H CDR3 encoded H3 domain are critical for the formation of the presumed "cavity-like" site in W3129 [90].

Several investigators using divergent immunization schemes have produced panels of mAb to B1355S and B512F dextran. In a panel where pure soluble B512F dextran was used for immunization of C57BL/6 mice, restriction to $V_H J558:V\kappa4$

family genes (73%) was observed [45]. Some heterogeneity in usage of J558 family genes, the largest V gene family in the mouse, was evident in that at least three V_H genes were used: $V_H45.21.1$, $V_H132.26$ and V_H102. A small subset of the panel used genes from other V_H families: V_HJ606 ($V_H22.1$) and V_HQ52 (V_HOx-1). In contrast, a mAb collection produced using adjuvants and multiple immunizations displayed a more heterogeneous distribution of V gene family usage (e.g., V_HJ558, $V_H36–60$, V_HX24 and V_HJ606; $V\kappa1$, $V\kappa2$, $V\kappa4$; [46, 48, 49]). Greater heterogeneity was evident among the specific V_HJ558 genes encoding these mAbs (e.g., V_H23, V_H6, $V_H45.21.1$, $V_H132.26$ and V_H102).

Abs elicited by TD dextran immunization also display heterogeneity in fine specificity. Immunization of mice with isomaltotriose (IM3)-KLH or isomaltohexaose (IM6)-KLH produce at least two separate fine specificities of antibodies which differ in the ability to bind IM3 (91). Spectrotype analysis of the serum from IM6-KLH immunized CBA and C57BL mice reveals a complex pattern, probably reflecting a diverse Ab response but all of the antibodies bound dextran. CBA mice are able to produce anti-dextran Abs when immunized with IM3-KLH while C57BL mice lacked the ability to produce anti-dextran Abs following IM3-KLH immunization. This strain difference mapped to the Igh locus, reflecting the absence of a V_H allele in C57BL mice. Among the antibodies produced by IM oligosaccharide–CSA immunization of BALB/c and C57BL mice are a subset of cavity-type mAbs using V_HX24:$V\kappa1$ [92]. Thus, like the TI-2 response, the TD response to dextran is complex and appears to recognize several fine specificities.

Serum Abs raised in BALB/c mice against B1355S dextran are mostly IgM:λ [93]. This response is strain specific; it is absent in CBA and C57BL mice and appears to map to the Igh locus. A panel of 10 IgM:λ mAbs produced in B1355S immunized BALB/c mice was similar to J558 and MOPC104E myeloma proteins in that they were V_HJ558:V_λ [47]. Heterogeneity in V_H somatic mutation and J_H segment usage were evident, which correlated with placement in 5 reactivity groups defined by quantitative precipitin analysis [94]. However, sequence comparison to the known germline V_H regions revealed that they were all most closely related to the same germline gene that encodes the J558 and M104E myelomas, $V_H45.21.1$. Immunization of BALB/c mice with nigerose–KLH elicits κ-chain serum antibodies, defining a separate specificity of $\alpha(1 \rightarrow 3)$ dextran reactive Abs [95]. Nigerose, unlike B1355S dextran, is pure $\alpha(1 \rightarrow 3)$ dextran, thus these Abs differ from the B1355S specific Abs in both fine specificity and V_L usage. CAL20 TEPC1035, specific for B1355S dextran, is also a κ-isotype Ab [87].

In summary, a restricted set of V_H:V_L pairs dominate Ab responses to simple environmental PS such as levan, galactan and dextran, although minor pairing are also elicited (Table 1). These Abs tend to have moderate avidity and limited somatic mutation. In some instances, there is recurrent use of a V_H gene or family in Abs with a broad specificity (e.g., V_HJ558 in anti-dextran Abs, V_HJ606 in anti-levan Abs), while fine specificity is determined by V_L usage (dextran B512F, $V_\kappa4$; dextran B1355S, $V_\lambda1$; In$^+$ levan, $V_\kappa11$; In$^-$ levan, V_λ).

III. CAPSULAR PS

Some bacteria and fungi are surrounded by a PS capsular layer which serves both as a virulence factor and a target for host antibody responses (reviewed in

[96–98]). Capsular synthesis requires the coordinate action of several genes, and is often induced by environmental factors. The potential combinations of sugars, linkages, branch structures and potential chemical substitutions leads to a great diversity in capsular types. For example in *E. coli* alone, 80 capsular serotypes have been described [99]. Despite the type specificity, there is sharing of capsular PS structures between bacteria. For example, *E. coli* K1 and *N. meningitidis* group B share $\alpha(2 \to 8)$-linked *N*-acetylneuraminic acid capsules [100]. Some gut flora bacteria and pathogens share capsular PS leading to "natural immunity" to some pathogens, presumably by cross-priming of anti-PS antibodies.

Ab responses to capsular PS (CP) are generally type specific and CP behave like TI-2 antigens. Anti-capsular responses in adults are oligoclonal in nature, e.g., V region usage is diverse on the population level, but within individuals a small number of clonotypes are expressed. Antibody responses in infants are poor; immunization with pure PS vaccines affords little protection against encapsulated pathogens. Infants and very young children are particularly susceptible to infections of encapsulated bacteria because there is a time lag between when maternal antibodies wane and when the TI-2 stimulated "natural immunity" antibodies arise. The idea to increase immunogenicity of capsular PS by conjugation to protein carriers was originally proposed 70 years ago [101]. Extensive research grounded in this initial observation has led to the development and introduction of PS-conjugate vaccines for infants, a major public health advance of the last ten years.

Haemophilus influenzae

H. influenzae is a gram-negative coccobacillus. Both unencapsulated and encapsulated strains (serotypes a–f) have been isolated, with *H. influenzae* type b (Hib) being the most common invasive form. Individuals over the age of five appear to be protected from Hib disease by the appearance of natural anti-PS antibodies which can be produced in response to carriage of Hib or other bacteria with cross-reactive capsular Ags (e.g., *E. coli* K100; [102]). The Hib CP is polymeric 3-β-D-ribose-$(1 \to 1)$-D-ribitol-5-phosphate (PRP, [103]). Passive administration of anti-Hib CP Abs has been demonstrated to confer protective immunity to invasive Hib disease [104].

Human immune responses to Hib CP are oligoclonal in nature, e.g., only a limited set of clonotypes are expressed in each individual [105]. Interestingly, Abs produced in response to infection or immunization with pure PS or conjugate vaccines differ in titer, but not in the oligoclonal nature [106–109]. Immunization with conjugate vaccines produces a memory response, but unlike other secondary responses, these appear to consist of expansion of existing clonotypes [108, 110].

While responses vary between individuals, predominant $V_H:V_L$ pairs are used. The majority of heavy chains are $V_H III$ [111, 112], mostly $V_H 3$–23, $V_H 3$–15 and $V_H 3$–49 [113, 114]. In most individuals the dominant response includes $V_\kappa II$ Abs, encoded by the A2 gene and detectable with an anti-idiotype reagent, HibId-1 (115, 116). The L3 loop structure of the A2 Abs appears to be critical for Ag binding. The CDR3 is invariably 10 amino acids in length, and contains a conserved Arg at 95a [117]. Substitutions (except R95aK) at this position reduce avidity, particularly substitutions to negatively charged amino acids (e.g., R95aE, R95aD; [22]). Other light chain clonotypes also are expressed ($V_\kappa I$, O2, O8/18, L11; $V_\kappa II$, A1/A17; $V_\kappa III$, A27; $V_\kappa IV$, B3; V_λ, 1–4, 3–3) in subsets of patients [118–120], including light-chains common in auto-antibodies (e.g., $V_\kappa A27$; [120]). Strikingly, a large subset of the anti-Hib CP, non-A2 light-chains also possess Arg residues at the VJ junction [119].

Functional differences between A2 responses and non-A2 responses have been described. Unlike the A2 Abs, the other clonotypes are cross-reactive with *E. coli* K100 PS (polymeric 3-β-D-ribose-(1$\rightarrow$2)-D-ribitol-5-phosphate (105, 121)), and contain more somatic mutations [118]. In contrast, the A2 Abs are higher avidity, and possess more *in vitro* bactericidal activity [109]. The absence of the A2 gene in members of some Native American populations may explain their higher incidence of *Haemophilus* disease [122]. Vaccination strategy also impacts Ab functional activity. Prp-OMP makes a lower avidity Ab response with a higher proportion of Abs recognized by a second anti-Id reagent specific for $V_\lambda VII$ light chains, HibId-2 [123]. In addition, HibId-1$^+$ Abs elicited by HibPS-OMP are lower avidity, and possess less bactericidal activity [124]. The fact that the Prp-OMP vaccine still affords protection argues that the threshold level of Abs or immune memory needed for protection can be achieved even with sub-optimal immunization.

Neisseria meningitidis

N. meningitidis is a gram-negative diplococcus responsible for a significant portion of endemic and epidemic bacterial meningitis. *N. meningitidis* can cause invasive diseases such as otitis media or sepsis or merely colonize asymptomatic carriers. The attack rate of *Meningococcal* diseases is highest for children and infants, probably because they lack effective immunity to the capsular PS. Factors leading to epidemic *Meningococcal* disease include crowded living conditions, e.g., military barracks and college dormitories. At least a dozen serogroups have been defined, but the majority of disease is caused by serogroups A, B, C, Y and W135, depending on the geographic location. Group A strains largely cause the *Meningococcal* epidemics in sub-Saharan Africa, while groups B and C cause the majority of cases in developed countries [125]. Like the Hib CP, human Ab responses to *Meningococcal* CP are oligoclonal in nature [126]. However, group A *Meningococcal* CP appears to be an exception among bacterial CP in that it elicits immune responses with TD qualities. For example, human infants mount Ab responses to group A CP [127–129], and T-cells appear to play a role in modulating murine Ab responses to group A CP [130].

Group B

Meningococcal group B capsular PS (MBPS) is a linear homopolymer of $\alpha(2\rightarrow8)$-linked sialic acid [131]. This capsular PS is shared with *E. coli* K1 and has been observed to be relatively less immunogenic than other *Meningococcal* PS, producing lower avidity Abs [100]. Antigenic similarity between MBPS and mammalian brain components have been described [132], arguing that auto-antigen specific tolerance may explain the poor immune responses to MBPS.

Mice immunized with MBPS produce typical TI-2 responses in that mostly IgM Abs are produced and secondary immunization generally does not produce enhanced Ab levels [133]. Variable levels of IgG can be produced depending on the mouse strain. Autoimmune NZB mice immunized with live encapsulated MenB bacteria produce particularly high levels of IgG (134). An NZB mAb, 735, was isolated and identified as $V_HJ558:V\kappa1$ (V_HMVARG:Vκbb1; [135, 136]). This IgG mAb may be unique among anti-PS Abs in that it binds an extended helical segment of MBPS of at least 10 NeuAc residues [21].

A diverse set of fine specificities has been defined by panels of anti-MBPS mAbs produced by immunization with TD or derivitized MBPS. N-propionylation is a strategy developed to modify the structure of MBPS and possibly lower the level of autoantigen cross-reactive antibodies [137]. Fine specificity distinctions drawn from MBPS Abs include specificity of mAbs raised against N-propionylated MBPS for short or long segment N-propionylated MBPS [137], degree of cross-reactivity of mAbs raised against N-acetyl MBPS to *E. coli* K92 PS [138], and degree of cross-reactivity of anti-short segment mAbs raised against N-propionylated MBPS to N-acetyl MBPS or inhibition by oligosaccharides [139]. In some instances, fine specificity differences correlated with functional activity. Pon *et al.* [137] demonstrated that mAbs specific for extended helical segment MBPS (> 10 sialic acids) had greater *in vitro* bactericidal activities. In another panel of 10 mAbs, a fraction of mAbs with increased *in vitro* bactericidal activity possessed a fine specificity to a "hidden epitope" attained when MBPS was complexed with proteins [140]. Devi *et al.* [140] hypothesized that hidden epitopes on MBPS attained a stable accessible configuration when complexed to protein carriers and that this minority epitope was preferentially recognized by the immune system in an otherwise poorly immunogenic molecule.

Human immune responses to MBPS have similarly diverse $V_H:V_L$ pair usage. At least two $V_H:V\kappa$ pairs are used, V_HIIIb:VκI (V_H3–15:VκO2) and V_HIIIa:VκI, as demonstrated by sequence analysis of Abs from Epstein–Barr Virus (EBV) transformed B-cells [141, 142]. Additional heterogeneity of V_L usage has been identified by analysis of MBPS binding paraproteins and macroglobulins. The first described was NOV, a V_H IIIa:V_λII IgM macroglobulin (V_H3–7:V_λ1–7; [143, 144]). In a subsequent screen of 359 human paraproteins, ~2% were shown to possess MBPS reactivity. The 7 MBPS-reactive paraproteins found in the screen were further characterized for V_L usage, four are K and 3 are λ [145].

Group C

The CP of *Meningococcal* group C, MCPS, is a linear homopolymer of $\alpha(2 \rightarrow 9)$-linked sialic acids that are O-acetylated at carbons 7 and/or 8 [131]. Native MCPS has an average of 1.16 equivalents of O-acetyl per sialic acid (146).

Serum responses to MCPS in mice are largely IgM and IgG3 while immunization with TD MCPS conjugates (MCPS-tetanus toxoid) will elicit other γ-isotypes, elevated serum bactericidal activity and immune memory [147]. Like other PS, the ability to mount an anti-MCPS response develops with age [148, 149]. Panels of mAbs generated from MCPS and MCPS-TT immunized BALB/c mice revealed a heterogeneous usage of $V_H:V_L$ combinations [30, 150]. Greater than one half of the mAbs in both the MCPS (8/16) and MCPS-tetanus toxoid (TT); (15/23) panels were V_HJ558, the largest V_H family in the mouse, and all mAbs had K-chains. Clonotype restrictions were evident in that V_H3609 mAbs were represented only among mAbs generated against MCPS, while the MCPS-TT groups contained V_H7183 and V_HVGAM3-8 mAbs. MAb from mice immunized with pure PS contained fewer presumed somatic mutations than those from mice immunized with TT conjugate [151].

Five fine specificity groups were defined based on cross-reactivity *to E. coli* K92 PS (alternating $\alpha(2\rightarrow9)$ and $\alpha(2\rightarrow8)$ sialic acid) and non-*O*-acetylated MCPS (OAc$^-$). These groups were: mAbs reactive with native MCPS only; MCPS and OAc$^-$ reactive (OAc$^- \approx$ MCPS); MCPS and OAc$^-$ reactive (OAc$^- >$ MCPS), MCPS and OAc$^-$ reactive (OAc$^- <$ MCPS); and MCPS, OAc$^-$ and K92 reactive. A trend linking fine specificity and V_H gene usage was evident. For example, all three V_H3609 mAbs were native MCPS specific. In contrast, V_HJ558 mAbs were present in all five fine specificity groups. V_HJ558 is the largest V gene family and sequence analysis reveals that at least four V_HJ558 genes are used, and that the fine specificity groups differ in usage of individual V_HJ558 and Vκ genes [151]. Also, three different gene families (V_HX24, V_HJ558 and V_H7183) were represented in the four mAbs cross-reactive with K92. Similar V_H usage heterogeneity was seen in B-Cells from MCPS immunized humans and hu-PBMC-SCID mice isolated using anti-Id antibodies [152].

Streptococcus species

Streptococcus sp. comprise a large group of gram-positive cocci that includes harmless commensals as well as virulent pathogens. The Lancefield serological classification scheme was developed to differentiate β-hemolytic species [153].

Group A

Group A *Streptococcus* (*S. pyogenes*) is implicated in a high frequency of pharyngeal infections and plays a role in triggering autoimmune rheumatic fever and glomerulonephritis. Furthermore, infections of lysogenic group A streptococcus can cause scarlet fever if the infection results in an accumulation of pyrogenic toxins [125]. Hyaluronic acid, the group A capsular PS (GAC), is composed of alternating residues of *N*-acetyl-D-glucosamine and glucoronic acid. *N*-acetyl-D-glucosamine is the immuno-dominant epitope in antibody responses [154].

Murine anti-group A Ab responses were initially demonstrated to be heterogeneous by isoelectric focusing (IEF) analysis and reactivity with anti-Id antibodies (V_κ1^{GAC}, Id5, Id20, IdX; [24, 155, 156]), although ~50% of the response was V_κ1^{GAC+} [155]. Subsequent analysis of DNA rearrangements in a panel of 29 A/J hybridomas suggested that the anti-GAC response used at least two V_H genes (termed V_H9, V_H39) and four V_L genes (termed V_κ25-39, V_κ25-47, V_κ24A-8, and V_κ2-91; [157]). However, when the reported hybridoma sequences are compared to the currently known mouse germline V genes, the complexity diminishes. The V regions originally identified as V_κ25-39, V_κ25-47 and V_κ24A-8 are actually the V_κ24 family genes he24 and hf24 [158]. The V gene termed V_κ2-91 is actually the V_κ2 gene bd2, while the V genes termed V_H9 and V_H39 are actually both V_HJ606 (V_H22.1). Similar domination by V_HJ606 was evident in a separate panel of 26 A/J

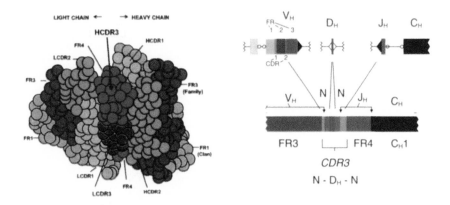

Plate 1. Location and generation of HCDR3. (A) A cartoon of the classic antigen binding site as seen head-on illustrates the central location of HCDR3. (B). HCDR3 is created by VDJ joining and N addition (reviewed in [2]). By virtue of the mechanisms that create it and the position it occupies, HCDR3 is the key to the diversification of the pre-immune repertoire. (See Figure 1, p. 44)

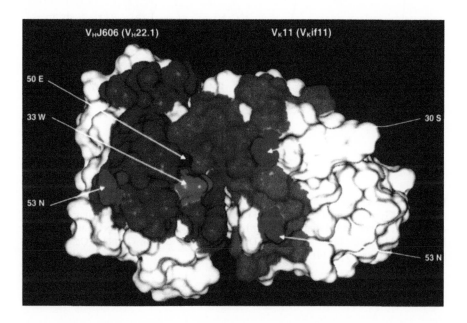

Plate 2. Molecular model of inulin binding mAb. Solvent accessible surface representation of the germline $V_H J606:V_K 11$ V region was constructed using the homology module of insight II 97.2 and the resolved PDB structures 1IAI (V_H), 1FVD (V_K) and 1NSN (H3 loop; description of method is in [62]). The FR surface is colored white; the CDR surface green. Residues demonstrated by site directed mutagenesis studies to be involved in inulin binding are red [62], while Trp33H, suggested by fluorescence binding experiments to contact Ag, is colored ochre [53]. (See Figure 1, p. 77)

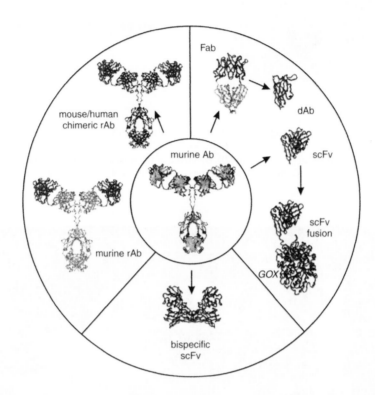

Plate 3. Forms of a recombinant antibodies (rAbs) shown as ribbon diagrams, derived from a murine IgG$_1$ monoclonal (center). (Fab) Fragment antigen binding; (scFv) single chain Fv antibody fragment; (dAb) diabody; (GOX) glucose oxidase. Images were generated using Insight II (Molecular Simulations, San Diego, CA) on a Silicon Graphics Octane workstation. (See Figure 1, p. 114)

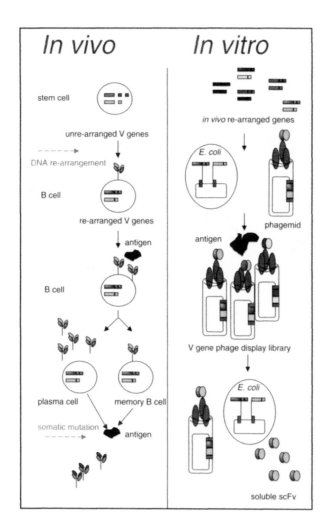

Plate 4. Comparison of *in vitro* phage-display libraries with the *in vivo* immune system. (See Figure 2, p. 119)

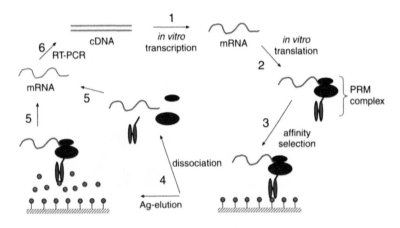

Plate 5. Ribosome display technology for the selection of rAb fragments. (See Figure 3, p. 129)

anti-GAC mAbs [159]. In this panel, the V_H22.1 CDR1 regions contained a concentration of presumed somatic mutations. A minority fraction of λ-isotype antibodies are also produced in mice immunized with GAC [155]. Thus, at least three V_H:V_L family pairs contribute to the anti-group A *Streptococcus* response; V_HJ606:$V_κ$2, V_HJ606:$V_κ$24 and a $V_λ$ combination.

In adult humans, unimmunized sera contain ~10 IEF bands reactive with GAC, indicative of limited clonal diversity [160]. Most Abs are IgG2, and clonotype expansion during ontogeny and clonotype shift following infection occur in the human anti-GAC repertoire.

Group B

Group B *Streptococcus* (*S. agalactiae*) is the most common cause of neonatal meningitis and sepsis in developed countries [125]. Several capsular types (e.g., Ia, Ib, and II–VI) cause disease, with type Ia serotype infections being the most common in early onset disease (shortly after birth) and type III in later onset disease [96, 161, 162]. Maternally derived anti-capsular antibodies are involved in neonatal protection [163]. Conjugate vaccines are under development for several serotypes [164–167].

Studies analyzing the antibody response to group B PS include two examinations of panels of mAbs. In one panel of 32 murine mAbs directed against type III PS, two fine specificities were identified; non-sialated PS and complete PS [168]. A second panel of 18 anti-type Ia and III Abs were produced by transformation of human lymphocytes with EBV but no heterogeneity was noted when two of these Abs were compared [169]. Unfortunately, there are no sequence data available for these Abs. An analysis of unimmunized donor sera provided evidence of limited clonotype (~15 IEF bands) and avidity variation in natural anti-type III Abs [170]. The individuals in this study had between two and six anti-type III clonotypes. Interestingly, like MBPS, anti-type III PS Abs appears to recognize an extended helical conformational epitope [171].

S. pneumoniae

S. pneumoniae (*Pneumococcus*) includes at least 90 serologically defined encapsulated strains. Virulence varies with capsular type and 23 strains cause the majority of *Pneumococcal* disease in industrialized countries. *Pneumococcal* diseases range from minor respiratory infections to potentially life-threatening pneumonia and meningitis. Infants and the elderly are particularly susceptible to *Pneumococcal* disease, and antibiotic resistant strains are emerging as a threat [172]. Carriage is common in healthy individuals and *Pneumococcal* disease often results from extension of nasopharyngeal colonization to adjacent structures [125].

Current *Pneumococcal* PS vaccines consist of mixtures of the capsular PS from each of the 23 disease causing strains [96] and the recently approved seven valent conjugate vaccine [173]. Immune responses to the phosphorylcholine (PC) epitope of the pan-Pneumococcal C-polysaccharide [174] also have been proposed to be involved in host protection [175, 176]. This contention is controversial [177, 178] in part because electron microscope (EM) studies have suggested that capsular PS likely conceals the C-polysaccharide from the immune system [179].

Mice immunized with *Pneumococcal* PS produce type-specific Abs, but there is some overlap of epitopes between closely related serotypes (e.g., 19A and 19F, [180]; 9A, 9L, and 9V, [181]). Protein conjugates are able to induce enhanced γ-isotype Ab responses to serotype 9V in neonatal mice [182].

Adult human immune responses to *Pnuemococcal* PS are oligoclonal in nature in that Abs are limited to 1–3 clones in individual patients [183, 184]. In contrast, heterogeneity in the Ab response is evident at the population level, responses involve both K- and λ-Abs, and extensive V region usage is evident [185, 186]. For some serotypes, biased, but not exclusive, V_H region usage may be evident (e.g., V_H3 with serotype 6B; [186]). In other instances, a bias toward K over λ-chain expression has been observed (e.g., serotype 23F; [183]). Ab avidity to 6B and 23F PS appears to correlate with protective efficacy against bacteremia when antibodies are transferred into mice [187]. As in mice, conversion of *Pneumococcal* PS to TD protein conjugate forms significantly enhances expression of γ-isotypes in adult humans [188].

Infant responses to most *Pneumococcal* PS (e.g., 6A, 18C and 19F) display classical features of anti-PS responses in that Ab responses are poor. The exception appears to be serotype three *Pneumococcal* PS, where a strong IgG Ab response can be induced as early as two months of age [189, 190]. Conjugate forms of other *Pneumococcal* PS (e.g., 6B, 14, 18C, 19F, 23F) induce γ-isotype responses in infants [191], including enhanced opsonizing antibodies to at least one serotype, 6B [192]. In addition, boosting infants with conjugate forms after a primary conjugate immunization induces higher avidity antibodies than boosting with pure PS [193]. These serological parameters of immunity appear to correlate with protection in a large pediatric study, administration of a seven-valent *Pneumococcal* conjugate vaccine has shown efficacy in preventing invasive disease and diminishing prevalence of otitis media [173]. Saccharide chain length has an impact on immunogenicity in infants, with serotype 19F polysaccharide conjugates being more immunogenic than oligosaccharide conjugates [194]. The conjugate protein carrier also impacts the immunogenicity in human infants. Serotypes 6B and 23F PS CRM and TT conjugates induced Abs in infants with the higher avidity than DT or OMPC conjugates [195].

Cryptococcus neoformans

The encapsulated yeast *C. neoformans* is an opportunistic pathogen for immunocompromised individuals (e.g., AIDS patients [196]). Inhalation of fungi can result in a primary pulmonary infection, which in some instances disseminates to other sites such as the central nervous system. The *Cryptococcal* capsule is a mixture of three components; a PS glucuronoxylomannan (GXM) and two minor constituents, galactoxylomannan and mannoprotein [197]. GXM comprises about 88% of the capsular material and is a linear polymer of $(1\rightarrow3)$-α-D-mannopyranan with β-D-xylopyranosyl, β-D-glucopyranosyluronic acid, and 6-O-acetyl substituents. The degree of substitution divides GXM into at least 5 serotypes (A–D and A/D), with the majority of infections in AIDS patients being serotype A.

Murine immune responses to GXM use restricted in $V_H:V_L$ genes varying with capsular PS serotypes. In one panel of eight hybridomas from BALB/c mice infected with strain GH *Cryptococcus* (serotypes A/D or D), seven serotype D specific mAbs were $V_H X24/V_\lambda$ ($V_H Gal55.1$) and one identified as $V_H 7183/V\kappa 5.1$ ($V_H 50.1:V\kappa bb1$, [198]). The $V_H 7183/V\kappa 5.1$ mAb possessed a broader fine specificity in that it also bound serotype A PS. In contrast to group D Abs, all 29 Abs of panel from BALB/c mice either infected with serotype A *Cryptococcus* or immunized with type A GXM-TT were $V_H 7183/V\kappa 5.1$ [199]. A difference in the pattern of isotype expression was evident between infected and TD immunized mice in that infection produced IgM Abs while immunization elicited more IgG Abs. Most mAbs bound all four GXM types in the rank order of A > B > D > C. The exception was one mAb with a framework V_H substitution R38T and a higher affinity for C-GXM than D-GXM. Thus, in a manner similar to that observed in the $V_H 53$ substitution in inulin Abs, a single amino acid change resulted in a fine specificity shift in dual reactive Abs. NZB/W mice immunized with GXM-TT conjugates also produced mostly $V_H 7183:V\kappa 5.1$ Abs [200].

A range of $V_H:V_L$ combinations were used in mAbs generated from BALB/c and C3H/HeJ mice immunized by serotypes A, B, C and D PS-RBC conjugates [201], correlating with a variety of fine specificities. The BALB/c mAbs included two $V_H 10:V\kappa 21$ ($V_H MRL-DNA4:V\kappa hf24$), two $V_H VGAM:V\kappa 4/5$ ($V_H GK1A:V\kappa kk4$, $V_H GK1B:V\kappa kk4$), and two $V_H 7183:V\kappa 5.1$ ($V_H 7183.10:V\kappa bb1$, $V_H 69.1:V\kappa bb1$) mAbs. One C3H/HeJ mAb was identified as $V_H 11:V\kappa ser$ ($V_H 11:V\kappa 19-32$). Like the $V_H 7183/V\kappa 5.1$ mAbs of Mukherjee *et al.* [199], the $V_H 10/V\kappa 21$ mAbs bound multiple serotypes. The $V_H VGAM:V_\kappa 4/5$ mAbs were specific for serotypes A and D, and the $V_H 11:V\kappa ser$ mAb was serotype A specific. Based on the variable region gene usage, the available anti-*Cryptococcal* mAbs were divided into five groups (I, $V_H 11$; II, $V_H 7183$; III, $V_H 10$; IV, $V_H VGAM$; V, $V_H X24$). In a follow-up report using a slightly larger panel of mAbs, at least five GXM epitopes were defined based on reactivity patterns to GXM serotypes and an agreement was observed between the reactivity and V_H region groups [202].

Similarly restricted $V_H:V_L$ region usage was noted in two human mAbs from individuals immunized with GXM-TT. The mAbs were $V_H 3/V_\lambda 1a$ ($V_H 3-23:V_\lambda 1-19$ and $V_H 3-7:V_\lambda 1-19$). The VH gene difference translated into a fine specificity difference, the $V_H 3-7$ mAb bound serotypes A, B and D, while the $V_H 3-23$ mAb other all serotypes [203].

Other Gram-negative Bacteria

Anti-capsular or exo-polysaccharide antibodies are involved in host protection against other gram-negative bacteria, although the degree of characterization of their genetics and immunology are less comprehensive than Hib and *Meningococcus*. Confounding factors for analyses of anti-capsular responses to other gram-negative bacteria include the observations that often anti-LPS antibodies may be more important for host protection [204] or that encapsulation is not a requisite for virulence (e.g., *V. cholerae* serotypes O1 vs. O139, *E. coli* O157:H7; [205, 206]).

Salmonella typhi

S. Typhi is the cause of typhoid fever, an invasive enteric and systemic infection. *S. typhi* is surrounded by a PS capsule layer, termed Vi, a linear homopolymer of α(1→ 4)-*O*-acetyl-*N*-acetyl-galactosaminuronic acid [207]. Immunization of mice with Vi elicits antibodies specific for at least two Vi epitopes defined by cross-reactivity between *Salmonella* and *Citrobacter* Vi. One panel of anti-Vi mAb, containing both κ and λ mAbs, bound both *Salmonella* and *Citrobacter* Vi antigen [208]. In contrast, a second panel of 4 IgM mAb from BALB/c mice immunized with *S. typhi* recognized *Salmonella* Vi but not *Citrobacter* Vi antigen [209]. Finally, mAbs reactive with non-*O*-acetylated Vi have been described [210], adding additional heterogeneity to the anti-Vi response. Human immune responses to Vi antigen appear to be TI-2 in nature, prompting the design of conjugate Vi vaccines which have elicit Ab responses with higher titers in 2–4 year old children than pure PS vaccines [211].

Pseudomonas aeruginosa

P. aeruginosa is a cause of nosocomial infections and opportunistic pulmonary infections in cystic fibrosis (CF) patients. Mucoid strains of *P. aeruginosa*, those that infect CF patients, secrete muco-exopolysaccharide (MEP) as a virulence factor. MEP, which varies between strains, consists of polymers of β(1→ 4) linked mannuronic and guluronic acid [212]. At least two serological epitopes have been defined on MEP; one common epitope on MEP of all mucoid strains and one epitope shared only by strains 1 and 258 [212]. Differences in *in vitro* functional activity (e.g., opsonization) of anti-MEP Abs also have been linked to the V region of the antibodies, presumably reflecting differences in fine specificity or avidity [213]. Whether these *in vitro* functional differences translate into delayed colonization of CF patients with *Pseudomonas* and altered courses of disease is controversial [214, 215].

Escherichia coli

E. coli are a group of enteric coccobacilli strains that encompass both normal gut flora and virulent pathogens. A broad range of capsular types have been identified, including some implicated with urinary tract infections (e.g., K1; [99]). *E. coli* that lack capsules have also been identified, including highly virulent strains (e.g., O157:H7; [205]). Because of the number of CP types (K antigens), there is some sharing of antigenic determinants. For example, immunization of mice with K92 PS ((2→8)-α-N-acetylneuraminic acid-(2→9)NeuNAc) not only induces Abs to K92 PS but also MCPS ((2→ 9)NeuNAc) and the poorly immunogenic K1 PS ((2→8)NeuNAc; [216]). Protection against *E. coli* by anti-capsular sera or monoclonal antibodies has been demonstrated experimentally [217, 218]. Co-administration of anti-K1 capsular and anti-LPS mAbs have been demonstrated to afford greater protection than either alone, arguing for the utility of broadly reactive antibody responses [218]. Interestingly, a K5, but not a K1 capsule, inhibits the protective capacity of the anti-LPS mAb [218]. Thus, antibodies that target the outermost surface of *E. coli* appear to be the most effective for protection, and capsular type can influence the effectiveness of anti-LPS Abs.

Klebsiella pneumoniae

Like *E. coli*, *K. pneumoniae* has a diverse range of capsular types (K antigens; [219]), leading to diversity in human anti-K antigen Ab responses. In a set of eight mAbs generated from volunteers vaccinated with a 24 valent *Klebsiella* CP vaccine, seven fine specificities for serogroups were defined with each mAb specific for determinants shared by common clusters of serotypes [220]. Abs to the capsular components have been demonstrated to protect mice from experimental challenges of encapsulated *K. pneumoniae* [221, 222]. Anti-LPS Abs also are protective against *K. pneumoniae* challenges, but high doses of mAb are required to protect against encapsulated strains, presumably because the CP layer partially inhibits opsonophagocytosis [223]. As in *E. coli*, the degree of inhibition varies with capsular strain; K2 CP appears to be more effective at blockade of opsonophagocytosis than K7 or K21 CP [224].

IV. MAMMALIAN CELL SURFACE CARBOHYDRATES

Abnormal patterns of glycosylation on proteins and lipids have been shown to be associated with transformation (reviewed in [225]). A range of carbohydrate structures on glycosphingolipids has been defined. These carbohydrates have been sorted into three categories based on the core structure: the globoseries, the lactoseries and the ganglioseries. A large number of mAbs specific for carbohydrates from all three series have been raised, largely by injection of mice with human tumor cell lines. Most of these mAbs bind terminal saccharides of the glycolipids or glycoproteins, which are often galactose/galactosamine co-terminated with fucose or neuraminic acid. Because the field is more concerned with generation of tumor–lytic mAbs than PS immunology, only one or a small number of mAbs are produced at a time, and variable region sequence and epitope information are not always available. However, some studies of the diversity of V gene usage in cell surface Abs have been performed. These studies indicate that partial V region genetic restriction also occurs in these antibody responses, although more extensive somatic mutation was evident in auto-antigen specific paraproteins isolated from patients.

Fucosyllactosamine

Antibodies to 3-fucosyllactosamine (FL, CD15, Le^x) have demonstrated genetic restriction depending on their derivation history. A panel of seven IgM mAbs raised in mice against FL were all V$_H$X24:Vκ24B (V$_H$Gal55.1:Vκhe24), with some somatic mutations [226]. In contrast, high affinity phage display library Abs differed from the murine mAbs in both V$_L$ usage and fine specificity [227]. Although they used the same V$_H$X24 gene, they had different D (DSP2.9 and PFL16.2 vs. Q52) and J$_H$ (3 and 4 vs. 4) gene segments. The light chain variable regions were also markedly different in Vκ (Vκce9 and Vκkk4 vs. Vκhe24) and Jκ (2 and 4 vs. 1) usage, as was fine specificity (also binding sialated Le^x and nLc4Cer). Moreover, FL reactive paraproteins present in human sera were heterogeneous in light chain usage (κ vs. λ) and fine specificity (FL alone vs. also binding sialated Le^x and nLc4Cer; [228]). Thus, while one V$_H$:V$_L$ pair predominates in anti-FL Abs produced in an artificial murine system, more diverse responses to FL are possible.

Gangliosides and Globosides

Trends towards genetic restriction in murine Ab responses to gangliosides and globosides have been described. In one study, a panel of nine mAbs was generated against disialogangliosides (GD2, GD3) by immunization of BALB/c and A/J mice with whole tumor cells, purified GD3 or O-acetyl-GD3 gangliosides [229]. This panel contained Abs with diverse variable regions and fine specificities, but five of the nine were V_HJ558. In a more comprehensive northern blot screen of 46 murine anti-ganglioside mAbs generated in multiple labs, trends toward genetic restriction of V_H gene usage were evident despite variation in immunization strategies [230]. MAbs specific for NeuAcα(2→3) or (2→8) linkages (e.g., GM2, GD2) tended to use V_HJ558 (71%), as did mAbs specific for sulfated glycolipids (80%). MAbs specific for NeuAcα(2→6) linkages used V_HQ52 (5 mAbs) and mAbs specific for NeuAcα(2→9) linkages used V_HJ606 (3 mAbs). Genetic restriction has been noted also in anti-galactosylgloboside (GalGb4, SSEA-3 antigen) antibodies. Four mAbs produced against this Ag are $V_HX24:V_KOx-1$ ($V_HGal55.1:V_Kai4$; [231]), providing another example of a $V_HGal55.1$ anti-PS specificity. Mutation of 99Tyr of V_H of one of these antibodies ablates binding to GalGb4 [232], providing another example of an aromatic amino acid critical for PS:Ig interactions [41, 53, 62].

A lesser degree of genetic restriction has been noted in anti-ganglioside Abs isolated as EBV transformants from autoimmune patients. In a panel of three mAb reactive to GD2 and GD3, restriction to $V_HIII:V_KIV$ was noted ($V_H3-23:V_KB3$; [233]). An individual human mAb with a broad GD3, GM3 and GD2 reactivity also used V_HIII, but paired with VκII ($V_H3-23:V_KA17$; [234]). A complicated picture of genetic restriction was found in anti-GM1 mAbs. In one set of ten motor neuropathy mAbs, no bias towards genetic restriction of either V_H or V_L was noted [31]. In a second set of motor neuropathy mAbs [32], a bias towards V_HIII usage was noted (five of six clones used V_H3-30 or V_H3-7), while V_L region usage was variable (VκC6, $V_λ1-16$, $V_λ3-4$, $V_λ1-3$, $V_λ1-4$). Extensive somatic mutation was apparent in Abs from both studies, as well as heterogeneity of fine specificity (e.g., anti-GM1 vs. also binding asialo-GM1 and GD1b). Analysis of myeloma serum paraproteins reactive with GM1 also revealed heterogeneity of light chain usage and fine specificity [228]. The small number of available human ganglioside reactive mAbs [6–10] and the complex nature of the immunologic process behind their generation are confounding factors for these analyses. Nonetheless, some hint of bias towards certain V regions is evident.

Cold Agglutinins

The blood antigens i and I are comprised of repeating N-acetyl lactosamine attached to proteins or ceramides on RBC surfaces. Autoantibodies to these structures, termed cold agglutinins, can cause hemolysis and severe anemia. Panels of EBV transformants expressing cold agglutinins have been analyzed for V region usage. V_H4 (V_H4-34) is the predominant V_H region for both i and I [235, 236], while V_L usage is Ag specific. Anti-I Abs use VκIII (VκL2), while anti-i Abs use predominantly VκI (VκO2), together with VκIII and $V_λ$ in a minority of Abs [236]. As in anti-levan Abs (62), fine specificity in cold agglutinins is not determined solely by V_L, as transfer of H3 loops from anti-i Abs into anti-I Abs abrogates binding to the I antigen [237].

V. STRUCTURES OF ANTI-PS ABS

Insights into PS:Ig interaction are gradually being gained as resolved structures of anti-PS Abs and PS:Ig complexes accumulate. Antibody/antigen interactions are formed by complementarity between the antigen-binding CDR surface in the variable region of the antibody and the structure of the antigen (reviewed in [18]). Antigen binding involves multiple non-covalent interactions between atoms in the antigen and the CDR surface, although only about 1/3 to 1/5 of the CDR surface participates directly in antigen contact. In the three-dimensional structure of the variable regions, the residues in the CDR regions form loops, H1–3 in the heavy chain and L1–L3 in the light chain, between the strands of the β-pleated sheet of the immunoglobulin domain. Three-dimensional structural analysis has defined canonical structures for 5 of the 6 CDR loops, facilitating the prediction of the structure of antibodies for which the three-dimensional structure has not been resolved. The H3 loop has eluded classification, although some rules delineating its structure have been described.

Amino acids most crucial for antigen binding are in CDR regions, in many instances by the formation of contacts with the antigen (e.g., hydrogen bonds, salt-bridges, Van der Waals interactions). However, the relationship between antigen contact and affinity is complex in that some residues do not directly contact antigen, rather via interactions with water molecules [18, 238]. Sites outside of the CDRs also influence affinity, for example FR residues near the CDR region often contribute to the structure of the CDR surface. Structural changes to the CDR surface induced by antigen binding have been described in comparisons between resolved structures of free antibodies and antibody-antigen complexes.

The consistent appearance of the V_HGal55.1 (also termed V_H441) member of the V_HX24 family in anti-PS antibodies (Table I; $\alpha(1\rightarrow6)$ galactan, $\beta(2\rightarrow6)$ levan, *Cryptococcal* group D CP, FL, galactogloboside) has raised the suggestion that this gene has a natural tendency to bind PS, and that the light chain and DJ_H determine fine specificity. Based on a survey of Ab sequences, it has been reported that certain canonical hypervariable loop structures appear to favor PS specificities [16], raising the suggestion that V region restriction occurs to maintain a consensus PS binding surface topology.

Although only a handful of anti-PS Ab structures have been resolved, a few common characteristics can be observed after a systematic comparison [19–21, 74, 239–242]. First, aromatic residues such as Thr, Phe, Tyr, and His are often present in antigen contact portions of CDR surfaces of Abs specific for neutral PS. Secondly, conformational compatibility exists in CDR surface topography, e.g., the surface has pockets or depressions presumed able to accommodate sugars. A strict segregation of anti-PS surfaces into "cavity-type" and "groove-type" does not bear out, but Abs that bind terminal sugars have deeper pockets, similar to those predicted in structures of "cavity-type" antibodies. Shallower "groove-type" depressions are evident in other CDR surfaces, and some CDR surfaces have combinations of both features.

Individual Antibodies

A number of structures of anti-PS antibody Fab fragments have been resolved and in some cases modeling studies have predicted placement of the PS antigen in CDR binding surface. These modeling studies should be viewed with caution, given that antigen antibody binding can confer structural changes on both the

CDR surface of the antibody and the PS structure. For reference, we have provided a V gene identification and the PDB accession code for each structure (in parentheses, following the V gene pair identification).

The first anti-PS antibody to be resolved was the galactan binding J539 myeloma protein at 2.6Å (V_H55:Vκkb4; 2FBJ; [74]). The J539 binding site, predicted by earlier studies to bind a linear epitope of 4 α(1→6) linked galactans, was found to have a cavity-like structure with two grooves leading away from the cavity. The cavity is lined predominantly with aromatic amino acids (e.g., Trp 92L, Trp 33H, His 52H, Tyr 92L) with two additional Tyr residues on the outer surface (e.g., Tyr 101H, Tyr 104H). The two grooves are also partially lined with these same aromatic residues (e.g., Try 92L, Trp 33H, His 52H). Previous studies with Trp fluorescence changes predicted that both Trp 92L and Trp 33H are involved with antigen contact [41].

B72.3, an antibody that recognizes a combination PS/amino acid epitope, TAG72 (NeuAc2→6aGalNAcα1→O→Ser/Thr), has been resolved to 3.1 Å (V_H102:Vκ12–46; 1BBJ; [239]). The presumed binding site of this antibody has the form of a basket with a Tyr-rich (Tyr 96, Tyr 97) base. Packed alongside are V_L CDR residues Phe 91 and Tyr 96. Some of these residues (Tyr 96L), interact with internal residues via H bonds, but others are available to contact antigen (Tyr 97H).

The anti-*Cryptococcal* capsular mAb, 2H1, was resolved to 2.4Å ($V_H7183.10$:Vκb-b1; 2HIP; [240]). The binding site is in the form of a depression formed by residues from L3, H1, H2 and H3. Among the residues that form this depression are two aromatic amino acids, Trp 96L and Phe 33H. A Trp residue in a similar position in a related $V_H7183.10$:Vκbb1 mAb, mAb439, was demonstrated by fluorescence and acrylamide quenching studies to contact the cryptococcal capsular GXM PS [243].

The mAb735, specific for the negatively charged PS α(2→8) sialic acid (MBPS), has been resolved to 2.8 Å ($V_H102.1$:$V_κ$bb1; 1PLG; [21]). This antigen differs from other PS antigens in that its largely helical structure allows recognition of a relatively long epitope (10 sugars in length; [244]). The binding site of mAb735 differs from the antibodies that bind neutral PS in that the CDR surface has a relatively charged nature. One side of the binding site, formed largely by L3 and H2, is a convex surface displaying three positively charged residues, Lys 59H, Lys 65H and Lys 101H. The other side, formed largely by L2 and H3, is a relatively uncharged groove with two oppositely charged adjacent residues Asp 105H and Arg 98H. Modeling of α(2→8) sialic acid into the binding site predicts that all three Lys residues participate in salt bridges with antigen, and about 30 additional hydrogen bonds are formed between the PS and CDR surface. Thus, the overall positive charge of the CDR is predicted to contribute significantly to its specificity against a negatively charged PS.

The resolved structures of two anti-ganglioside antibodies have been reported recently by independent groups. The anti-GD2 ganglioside antibody, ME36.1, was resolved at a 2.8 Å resolution ($V_H45.21.1$:Vκap4; 1PSK; [241]). The binding site was found to have a shallow groove type structure (20 Å long × 10 Å wide × 8 Å deep) consistent with binding the PS chain of GD2. The total contact area of the site is a 413 Å^2, highly aromatic surface with four Phe and four Tyr residues (Phe 95L, Phe 97L, Phe 64H, Phe 101H, Tyr 93L, Tyr 32H, Tyr 60H, Tyr 95H). Strikingly, modeling studies do not predict extensive contacts between antigen and the aromatic residues.

An anti-GD3 ganglioside antibody, R24, and its chimeric counterpart, chR24, have been resolved to 3.1 Å and 2.5 Å (V_HMOPC21:$V_\kappa$cc9; 1R24; 1BZ7; [242]). The GD3 antigen differs from GD2 by one sugar residue, a branched N-acetylgalactosamine ($1 \rightarrow 4$) linked to the penultimate galactose in GD2. R24 possess a distinct fine specificity in that it is specific for GD3 while ME36.1 binds both GD2 and GD3, but with a much higher avidity for GD2. In contrast to ME36.1, R24 has a relatively deep pocket (8.5 Å × 12 Å × 8 Å), presumed to accommodate the terminal sialic acid of GD3. This pocket formed by the H1, H2, and H3 loops is lined with polar and aromatic amino acids, largely Ser, Thr, His and Tyr.

The *Fab* structure of KAU, a human IgM reactive with the cold agglutinin antigen I, has been resolved to 2.8 Å (1QLR; V_H4-34:VκA11; [245]). The KAU combining site topology is complex, composed of an extended cavity and a small pocket. Interestingly, loops associated with cold agglutinin restriction to V_H4-34 (H1, H2) comprise the pocket. In contrast, loops associated with I and i fine specificity distinction make up the cavity (H3, L1, L3; [235–237]). Both indentations contain some aromatic residues (Tyr 92L, Trp47H and Tyr33L in the cavity and His53H in the pocket), but a very striking feature is a predominance of Ser residues (94L, 93L, 30L, 31L surrounding the cavity, 54H and 56H surrounding the pocket).

PS:Ig Complexes

Currently, the two structurally resolved PS-Ig complexes are the Sel55-4 antibody complexed with the *Salmonella* O-antigen (1MFD; [20]), and BR96 antibody complexed with the Lewis Y antigen (Le^y; 1CLY; 1CLZ; [19]). The nature of the contacts between Ig and PS differ somewhat from those of other resolved protein: PS complexes in that there is a relative lack of involvement of stacking interactions between sugar and aromatic amino acid rings and no clear dominance of Asp, Asn and Glu residues in forming hydrogen bonds with PS [246].

The Sel55-4:O-antigen structure has been resolved to 2.05Å (V_H119.13:V_λ1; [20]). Sel55 binds a trisaccharide epitope, αD-Gal($1 \rightarrow 2$)[αD-Abe($1 \rightarrow 3$)]αD-Man of the O-antigen with relatively low affinity (2×10^5 M^{-1}). The 304 Å^2 binding site consists of both a shallow cavity (8 Å deep by 7 Å wide) and surface residues. The abequose branch side chain of the PS is accommodated by the shallow cavity, while the Man and Gal sugars lie perpendicular to the V_H:V_L interface. Thus, this antibody is neither "groove-type" nor "cavity-type", but a combination of both. Contact with antigen is dominated by H-bonds with aromatic residues (His 97H, His 35H, His 32L, Trp 95L, Trp 91L, Tyr 99H) and hydrophobic interactions. The H1, H3, L1 and L3 loops of the antibody participate in antigen contact, with about 60% of the contact surface comprised of V_H residues. A high degree of specificity of the antibody probably results in part from a buried water molecule that coordinates four hydrogen bonds with the abequose and the CDR surface, a sterically demanding interaction.

The BR96:Le^y complex has been resolved to 2.8 Å (V_H50.1:$V_\kappa$cr1 [19]). The CDR contact surface is 422 Å^2, with a large deep pocket (12 Å wide, 10 Å deep), and is largely comprised of V_H residues (79%). This pocket is lined with aromatic residues (Tyr 32L, Tyr 32H, Tyr 33H, Tyr 35H, Tyr 50H, Trp 100AH, Phe 96L, and His 27DL), and contacts between these residues and PS dominate binding. All four hexoses of Le^y are involved in CDR contacts, despite the relatively low affinity (2×10^5 M^{-1}) and the non-reducing end of the PS is buried in the CDR cavity, consistent with "cavity-type" binding.

VI. SUMMARY

In summary, extensive investigation has allowed some generalizations, with notable exceptions, about the nature of anti-PS Abs. A predominant feature of antibody responses to PS is genetic restriction. This is most obvious in responses to simple environmental PS such as galactan where only one V_H:V_L pair (V_HX24:V_κ4) is used. This genetic restriction and the frequent use of particular V genes (V_HGal55.1 for galactan, FL, levan, galactosylglobosides, *Cryptococcal* serotype D PS) has raised the suggestion that a consensus PS binding surface topology is selected for during B-cell responses. Further genetic restriction is evident in the isotypes used in anti-PS responses in that most are dominated by IgM and a restricted number of γ-isotypes (IgG3 in mice, IgG2 in humans). Isotype appears to impact the protectiveness of antibody responses, e.g., IgM antibodies appear to be more protective in a mouse model of Group B *Streptococcus* challenge than IgG antibodies. Antibody responses to more complex PS are more heterogeneous as demonstrated by the observations that antibody responses to capsular PS are oligoclonal and that greater V region heterogeneity can be generated in some instances with PS–protein conjugates.

Although PS have repeating structures and tend to have fewer epitopes than protein antigens, fine specificity differences can be demonstrated between Abs. Some Abs can be dual reactive, such as the J606 myeloma which binds both $\beta(2 \rightarrow 1)$ and $\beta(2 \rightarrow 6)$ levan. Fine specificity can be influenced by mutations in variable regions, such as in inulin-binding antibodies like J606 where mutations at V_H53 increases or decreases binding to $\beta(2 \rightarrow 1)$, but not $\beta(2 \rightarrow 6)$ levan. In other instances, such as cold agglutinins or globosides, V_H usage is restricted while the V_L appears to determine fine specificity.

Another predominant feature of anti-PS antibodies is moderate affinity. The evolution of antibody responses involves some degree of affinity maturation in that a few somatic mutations are evident in the panels of mAbs generated by immunization with simple PS, such as levan. A subset of these mutations have been demonstrated to affect increases in avidity. Often certain avidity increasing mutations are found recurrently in independent mAbs or myeloma proteins, suggesting that they are consistently selected for during affinity maturation. Autoantibodies to cell surface carbohydrates such as gangliosides possess more somatic mutations, reflecting the complex, but poorly understood, immunological process behind their generation.

Analysis of available anti-PS Ab structures have allowed some generalizations to be made about the nature of the PS binding CDR surface, but also added a degree of complexity. Complementarity between the CDR surface and PS has been noted, for example Abs that bind terminal saccharides tend to have deep pockets. However, a strict segregation between "groove-type" vs. "cavity type" CDR surfaces does not bear out. In general, the CDR surfaces suggested by earlier studies appear to be able to accommodate epitope sizes of 3–5 sugars. However, a clear exception exists in the case of Abs that bind helical PS such as MBPS and CP from Group B *Streptococcus* where the number of sugars required for the proper epitope conformation appears to be in excess of 10. In the two resolved structures of PS:Ig complexes (Sel55-4: *Salmonella* O-antigen and BR96:Le^y), hydrogen bonding between aromatic CDR amino acids and PS appear to dominate. Additional indirect evidence for a predominant role for aromatic V region amino acids in binding to neutral PS has also been provided by site directed mutagenesis (anti-inulin Abs) and fluorescence quenching studies (anti-galactan and levan Abs). In contrast, a basic CDR surface (e.g., Arg 95a in Hib Abs, MBPS Abs) appears to be critical for binding negatively charged PS.

ACKNOWLEDGMENTS

The authors would like to acknowledge the careful review of this manuscript by Drs. Marjorie Shapiro, Sean Fitzsimmons, and Carl Frasch.

REFERENCES

1. Stein, K.E. (1992). Thymus-independent and thymus-dependent responses to polysaccharide antigens. *J. Infect. Dis. 165 Suppl.* **1**, S49–52.
2. Sheehan, K.M., Mainville, C.A., Willert, S., and Brodeur, P.H. (1993). The utilization of individual VH exons in the primary repertoire of adult BALB/c mice. *J. Immunol.* **151**, 5364–5375.
3. Strohal, R., Helmberg, A., Kroemer, G., and Kofler, R. (1989). Mouse Vk gene classification by nucleic acid sequence similarity. *Immunogenetics* **30**, 475–493.
4. Potter, M., Newell, J.B., Rudikoff, S., and Haber, E. (1982). Classification of mouse VK groups based on the partial amino acid sequence to the first invariant tryptophan: impact of 14 new sequences from IgG myeloma proteins. *Mol. Immunol.* **19**, 1619–1630.
5. Kabat, E., Wu, T., Perry, H., Gottesman, K., and Foeller, C. (1991). Sequences of proteins of immunological interest. U.S. Department of Health and Human Services, National Institutes of Health, Bethesda, MD.
6. Altschul, S.F., Madden, T.L., Schaffer, A.A., Zhang, J., Zhang, Z., Miller, W., and Lipman, D.J. (1997). Gapped BLAST and PSI-BLAST: a new generation of protein database search programs. *Nucleic Acids Res.* **25**, 3389–3402.
7. Matsuda, F., Ishii, K., Bourvagnet, P., Kuma, K., Hayashida, H., Miyata, T., and Honjo, T. (1998). The complete nucleotide sequence of the human immunoglobulin heavy chain variable region locus. *J. Exp. Med.* **188**, 2151–2162.
8. Schable, K.F., and Zachau, H.G. (1993). The variable genes of the human immunoglobulin kappa locus. *Biol. Chem. Hoppe Seyler* **374**, 1001–1022.
9. Brensing-Kuppers, J., Zocher, I., Thiebe, R., and Zachau, H.G. (1997). The human immunoglobulin kappa locus on yeast artificial chromosomes (YACs). *Gene* **191**, 173–181.
10. Thiebe, R., Schable, K.F., Bensch, A., Brensing-Kuppers, J., Heim, V., Kirschbaum, T., Mitlohner, H., Ohnrich, M., Pourrajabi, S., Roschenthaler, F., Schwendinger, J., Wichelhaus, D., Zocher, I., and Zachau, H.G. (1999). The variable genes and gene families of the mouse immunoglobulin kappa locus. *Eur. J. Immunol.* **29**, 2072–2081.
11. Kawasaki, K., Minoshima, S., Nakato, E., Shibuya, K., Shintani, A., Schmeits, J.L., Wang, J., and Shimizu, N. (1997). One-megabase sequence analysis of the human immunoglobulin lambda gene locus. *Genome Res.* **7**, 250–261.
12. Tonegawa, S., Maxam, A.M., Tizard, R., Bernard, O., and Gilbert, W. (1978). Sequence of a mouse germ-line gene for a variable region of an immunoglobulin light chain. *Proc. Natl. Acad. Sci. USA* **75**, 1485–1489.

13. Bernard, O., Hozumi, N., and Tonegawa, S. (1978). Sequences of mouse immunoglobulin light chain genes before and after somatic changes. *Cell* **15**, 1133–1144.

14. Sanchez, P., Marche, P.N., Rueff-Juy, D., and Cazenave, P.A. (1990). Mouse V lambda x gene sequence generates no junctional diversity and is conserved in mammalian species. *J. Immunol.* **144**, 2816–2820.

15. Snapper, C.M., and Mond, J.J. (1996). A model for induction of T cell-independent humoral immunity in response to polysaccharide antigens. *J. Immunol.* **157**, 2229–2233.

16. Lara-Ochoa, F., Almagro, J.C., Vargas-Madrazo, E., and Conrad, M. (1996). Antibody-antigen recognition: a canonical structure paradigm. *J. Mol. Evol.* **43**, 678–684.

17. Boswell, C.M., and Stein, K.E. (1996). Avidity maturation, repertoire shift, and strain differences in antibodies to bacterial levan, a type 2 thymus-independent polysaccharide antigen. *J. Immunol.* **157**, 1996–2005.

18. Padlan, E.A. (1996). X-ray crystallography of antibodies. *Adv. Protein Chem.* **49**, 57–133.

19. Jeffrey, P.D., Bajorath, J., Chang, C.Y., Yelton, D., Hellstrom, I., Hellstrom, K.E., and Sheriff, S. (1995). The x-ray structure of an anti-tumour antibody in complex with antigen. *Nat. Struct. Biol.* **2**, 466–471.

20. Cygler, M., Rose, D.R., and Bundle, D.R. (1991). Recognition of a cell-surface oligosaccharide of pathogenic Salmonella by an antibody Fab fragment. *Science* **253**, 442–425.

21. Evans, S.V., Sigurskjold, B.W., Jennings, H.J., Brisson, J.R., To, R., Tse, W.C., Altman, E., Frosch, M., Weisgerber, C., Kratzin, H.D., and *et al.* (1995). Evidence for the extended helical nature of polysaccharide epitopes. The 2.8 A resolution structure and thermodynamics of ligand binding of an antigen binding fragment specific for alpha-(2->8)-polysialic acid. *Biochemistry* **34**, 6737–6744.

22. Lucas, A.H., Moulton, K.D., and Reason, D.C. (1998). Role of kappa II-A2 light chain CDR-3 junctional residues in human antibody binding to the Haemophilus influenzae type b polysaccharide. *J. Immunol.* **161**, 3776–3780.

23. Cisar, J., Kabat, E.A., Dorner, M.M., and Liao, J. (1975). Binding properties of immunoglobulin combining sites specific for terminal or nonterminal antigenic determinants in dextran. *J. Exp. Med.* **142**, 435–459.

24. Perlmutter, R.M., Hansburg, D., Briles, D.E., Nicolotti, R.A., and Davie, J.M. (1978). Subclass restriction of murine anti-carbohydrate antibodies. *J. Immunol.* **121**, 566–572.

25. Siber, G.R., Schur, P.H., Aisenberg, A.C., Weitzman, S.A., and Schiffman, G. (1980). Correlation between serum IgG-2 concentrations and the antibody response to bacterial polysaccharide antigens. *N. Engl. J. Med.* **303**, 178–182.

26. Rudikoff, S., Mushinski, E.B., Potter, M., Glaudemans, C.P., and Jolley, M.E. (1973). Six BALB-c IgA myeloma proteins that bind beta-(1–6)-D-galactan. Partial amino acid sequences and idiotypes. *J. Exp. Med.* **138**, 1095–1105.

27. Raff, H.V., Bradley, C., Brady, W., Donaldson, K., Lipsich, L., Maloney, G., Shuford, W., Walls, M., Ward, P., Wolff, E., and *et al.* (1991). Comparison of functional activities between IgG1 and IgM class-switched human monoclonal antibodies reactive with group B streptococci or Escherichia coli K1. *J. Infect. Dis.* **163**, 346–354.

28. Yuan, R., Casadevall, A., Spira, G., and Scharff, M.D. (1995). Isotype switching from IgG3 to IgG1 converts a nonprotective murine antibody to *Cryptococcus neoformans* into a protective antibody. *J. Immunol.* **154**, 1810–1816.

29. Wang, D., Wells, S.M., Stall, A.M., and Kabat, E.A. (1994). Reaction of germinal centers in the T-cell-independent response to the bacterial polysaccharide alpha(1->6)dextran. *Proc. Natl. Acad. Sci. USA* **91**, 2502–2506.

30. Garcia-Ojeda, P.A., Monser, M.E., Rubinstein, L.J., Jennings, H.J., and Stein, K.E. (2000). Murine immune response to *Neisseria meningitidis* group C capsular polysaccharide: analysis of monoclonal antibodies generated in response to a thymus-independent antigen and a thymus-dependent toxoid conjugate vaccine. *Infect. Immun.* **68**, 239–246.

31. Weng, N.P., Yu-Lee, L.Y., Sanz, I., Patten, B.M., and Marcus, D.M. (1992). Structure and specificities of anti-ganglioside autoantibodies associated with motor neuropathies. *J. Immunol.* **149,** 2518–2529.

32. Paterson, G., Wilson, G., Kennedy, P.G., and Willison, H.J. (1995). Analysis of anti-GM1 ganglioside IgM antibodies cloned from motor neuropathy patients demonstrates diverse V region gene usage with extensive somatic mutation. *J. Immunol.* **155,** 3049–3059.

33. Steinhoff, M. (1997). Haemophilus influenzae type b infections are preventable everywhere. *Lancet* **349,** 1186–1187.

34. Hadler, S., and Orenstein, W. (1997). *Principles and practices of pediatric infectious diseases.* Churchill – Livingstone, New York, New York.

35. Waldmann, T., and Nelson, D. (1995). Inherited Immunodeficiencies. In *Samter's immunologic diseases, vol.* Frank, I.M., Austen, K., Claman, H., and Unanue, E., eds. Little, Brown and Company, New York, New York, p. 387.

36. Wicker, L.S., and Scher, I. (1986). X-linked immune deficiency (xid) of CBA/N mice. *Curr. Top Microbiol. Immunol.* **124,** 87–101.

37. Potter, M., Mushinski, E.B., and Glaudemans, C.P. (1972). Antigen-binding IgA myeloma proteins in mice: specificities to antigens containing -D 1 leads to 6 linked galactose side chains and a protein antigen in wheat. *J. Immunol.* **108,** 295–300.

38. Rudikoff, S. (1988). Antibodies to beta(1,6)-D-galactan: proteins, idiotypes and genes. *Immunol. Rev.* **105,** 97–111.

39. Bos, N.A., Kimura, H., Meeuwsen, C.G., De Visser, H., Hazenberg, M.P., Wostmann, B.S., Pleasants, J.R., Benner, R., and Marcus, D.M. (1989). Serum immunoglobulin levels and naturally occurring antibodies against carbohydrate antigens in germ-free BALB/c mice fed chemically defined ultrafiltered diet. *Eur. J. Immunol.* **19,** 2335–2339.

40. Cebra, J.J., Gearhart, P.J., Halsey, J.F., Hurwitz, J.L., and Shahin, R.D. (1980). Role of environmental antigens in the ontogeny of the secretory immune response. *J. Reticuloendothel. Soc.* **28,** 61s–71s.

41. Glaudemans, C.P., Kovac, P., and Rasmussen, K. (1984). Mapping of subsites in the combining area of monoclonal anti-galactan immunoglobulin A J539. *Biochemistry* **23,** 6732–6736.

42. Bot, A., Nangpal, A., Pricop, L., Bogen, B., Kaushik, A., and Bona, C.A. (1996). V lambda-light chain genes reconstitute immune responses to defined carbohydrate antigens or haptens by utilizing different VH genes. *Mol. Immunol.* **33,** 1359–1368.

43. Boswell, C.M., Irwin, D.C., Goodnight, J., and Stein, K.E. (1992). Strain-dependent restricted VH and VL usage by anti-bacterial levan monoclonal antibodies. *J. Immunol.* **148,** 3864–3872.

44. Rudikoff, S., Rao, D.N., Glaudemans, C.P., and Potter, M. (1980). kappa Chain joining segments and structural diversity of antibody combining sites. *Proc. Natl. Acad. Sci. USA* **77,** 4270–4274.

45. Fernandez, C. (1992). Genetic mechanisms for dominant VH gene expression. The VHB512 gene. *J. Immunol.* **149,** 2328–2336.

46. Akolkar, P.N., Sikder, S.K., Bhattacharya, S.B., Liao, J., Gruezo, F., Morrison, S.L., and Kabat, E.A. (1987). Different VL and VH germ-line genes are used to produce similar combining sites with specificity for alpha(1–6)dextrans [published erratum appears in J Immunol 1987 Dec 1;139(11):3911]. *J. Immunol.* **138,** 4472–4479.

47. Clevinger, B., Schilling, J., Hood, L., and Davie, J.M. (1980). Structural correlates of cross-reactive and individual idiotypic determinants on murine antibodies to alpha-(1 leads to 3) dextran. *J. Exp. Med.* **151,** 1059–1070.

48. Wang, D.N., Chen, H.T., Liao, J., Akolkar, P.N., Sikder, S.K., Gruezo, F., and Kabat, E.A. (1990). Two families of monoclonal antibodies to alpha(1–6)dextran, VH19.1.2 and

VH9.14.7, show distinct patterns of J kappa and JH minigene usage and amino acid substitutions in CDR3. *J. Immunol.* **145**, 3002–3010.

49. Wang, D., Liao, J., Mitra, D., Akolkar, P.N., Gruezo, F., and Kabat, E.A. (1991). The repertoire of antibodies to a single antigenic determinant. *Mol. Immunol.* **28**, 1387–1397.

50. Carpita, N., Housley, T., and Hendrix, J. (1991). New features of plant-fructan structure revealed by methylation analysis and carbon-13 n.m.r. spectroscopy. *Carbohydrate Res.* **217**, 127–136.

51. Han, Y.W. (1990). Microbial levan. *Adv. Appl. Microbiol.* **35**, 171–194.

52. Lieberman, R., Potter, M., Humphrey, W., Jr., Mushinski, E.B., and Vrana, M. (1975). Multiple individual and cross-specific indiotypes on 13 levan-binding myeloma proteins of BALB/c mice. *J. Exp. Med.* **142**, 106–119.

53. Streefkerk, D.G., and Glaudemans, C.P. (1977). Binding studies on anti-fructofuranan mouse myeloma immunoglobulins A47N, A4, U61, and E109. *Biochemistry* **16**, 3760–3765.

54. Das, M., Streefkerk, D., and Glaudemans, C. (1979). The binding of inulo-oligosaccharides to homogeneous immunoglobulins E109 and A47N. *Mol. Immunol.* **16**, 97–100.

55. Vrana, M., Rudikoff, S., and Potter, M. (1978). Sequence variation among heavy chains from inulin-binding myeloma proteins. *Proc. Natl. Acad. Sci. USA* **75**, 1957–1961.

56. Vrana, M., Rudikoff, S., and Potter, M. (1979). The structural basis of a hapten-inhibitable kappa-chain idiotype. *J. Immunol.* **122**, 1905–1910.

57. Auffray, C., Sikorav, J., Ollo, R., and Rougeon, F. (1980). Correlation between D region structure and antigen binding specificity: evidence from the comparison of closely related immunoglobulin VH sequences. *Ann. Inst. Pasteur. Immunol.* **132D**, 77.

58. Streefkerk, D.G., Manjula, B.N., and Glaudemans, C.P. (1979). An interpretation of the apparent dual specificity of some murine myeloma immunoglobulins with inulinbinding activity. *J. Immunol.* **122**, 537–541.

59. Lieberman, R., Bona, C., Chien, C.C., Stein, K.E., and Paul, W.E. (1979). Genetic and cellular regulation of the expression of specific antibody idiotypes in the anti-polyfructosan immune response. *Ann. Immunol.* (Paris) **130**, 247–262.

60. Victor-Kobrin, C., Barak, Z.T., Bonilla, F.A., Kobrin, B., Sanz, I., French, D., Rothe, J., and Bona, C. (1990). A molecular and structural analysis of the VH and VK regions of monoclonal antibodies bearing the A48 regulatory idiotype. *J. Immunol.* **144**, 614–624.

61. Victor-Kobrin, C., Bonilla, F.A., Bellon, B., and Bona, C.A. (1985). Immunochemical and molecular characterization of regulatory idiotopes expressed by monoclonal antibodies exhibiting or lacking beta 2–6 fructosan binding activity. *J. Exp. Med.* **162**, 647–662.

62. Brorson, K., Thompson, C., Wei, G., Krasnokutsky, M., and Stein, K.E. (1999). Mutational analysis of avidity and fine specificity of anti-levan antibodies. *J. Immunol.* **163**, 6694–6701.

63. Brorson, K. Unpublished observations.

64. Gleeson, P.A., and Clarke, A.E. (1980). Antigenic determinants of a plant proteoglycan, the Gladiolus style arabinogalactan-protein. *Biochem. J.* **191**, 437–447.

65. Aspinall, G.O. (1969). Gums and mucilages. *Adv. Carbohydr. Chem. Biochem.* **24**, 333–379.

66. Manners, D.J., Pennie, I.R., and Ryley, J.F. (1973). The molecular structures of a glucan and a galactan synthesised by *Prototheca zopfii*. *Carbohydr. Res.* **29**, 63–77.

67. Glaudemans, C.P., Jolley, M.E., and Potter, M. (1973). Mammalian-lung galactan. *Carbohydr. Res.* **30**, 409–413.

68. Aspinall, G., Auret, B., and Hirst, E. (1958). Gum ghatti (Indian gum). Part III. Neutral oligosaccharides formed on partial acid hydrolysis of the gum. *J. Chem. Soc.* **221**, 4408–4414.

69. Ziegler, T., Pavliak, V., Lin, T.H., Kovac, P., and Glaudemans, C.P. (1990). Synthesis of specifically deoxygenated ligands related to (1–6)-beta-D-galacto-oligosaccharides, and

studies on their binding to monoclonal antigalactan antibodies. *Carbohydr. Res.* **204,** 167–186.

70. Ziegler, T., Kovac, P., and Glaudemans, C.P. (1990). A synthetic heptasaccharide reveals the capability of a monoclonal antibody to read internal epitopes of a polysaccharide antigen. *Carbohydr. Res.* **203,** 253–263.

71. Roy, A., Manjula, B.N., and Glaudemans, C.P. (1981). The interaction of two polysaccharides containing beta 1,6-linked galactopyranosyl residues with two monoclonal antigalactan immunoglobulin Fab' fragments. *Mol. Immunol.* **18,** 79–84.

72. Feldmann, R.J., Potter, M., and Glaudemans, C.P. (1981). A hypothetical space-filling model of the V-regions of the galactan-binding myeloma immunoglobulin J539. *Mol. Immunol.* **18,** 683–698.

73. Jolley, M.E., Rudikoff, S., Potter, M., and Glaudemans, C.P. (1973). Spectral changes on binding of oligosaccharides to murine immunoglobulin A myeloma proteins. *Biochemistry* **12,** 3039–3044.

74. Suh, S.W., Bhat, T.N., Navia, M.A., Cohen, G.H., Rao, D.N., Rudikoff, S., and Davies, D.R. (1986). The galactan-binding immunoglobulin Fab J539: an X-ray diffraction study at 2.6-A resolution. *Proteins* **1,** 74–80.

75. Glaudemans, C.P., Lerner, L., Daves, G.D., Jr., Kovac, P., Venable, R., and Bax, A. (1990). Significant conformational changes in an antigenic carbohydrate epitope upon binding to a monoclonal antibody. *Biochemistry* **29,** 10906–10911.

76. Hartman, A.B., and Rudikoff, S. (1984). VH genes encoding the immune response to beta-(1,6)-galactan: somatic mutation in IgM molecules. *Embo. J.* **3,** 3023–3030.

77. Steffan, W., Kovac, P., Albersheim, P., Darvill, A.G., and Hahn, M.G. (1995). Characterization of a monoclonal antibody that recognizes an arabinosylated (1->6)-beta-D-galactan epitope in plant complex carbohydrates. *Carbohydr. Res.* **275,** 295–307.

78. Knox, J., Linstead, P., Peart, J., Cooper, C., and Roberts, K. (1991). Developmentally regulated epitopes of cell surface arabinogalactan proteins and their relation to root tissue pattern formation. *Plant J.* **1,** 317–326.

79. Pennell, R.I., and Roberts, K. (1995). Monoclonal antibodies to cell-specific cell surface carbohydrates in plant cell biology and development. *Methods Cell Biol.* **49,** 123–141.

80. Menzies, A.R., Osman, M.E., Malik, A.A., and Baldwin, T.C. (1996). A comparison of the physicochemical and immunological properties of the plant gum exudates of *Acacia senegal* (gum arabic) and *Acacia seyal* (gum tahla). *Food Addit. Contam.* **13,** 991–999.

81. Jeanes, A. (1986). Immunochemical and related interactions with dextrans reviewed in terms of improved structural information. *Mol. Immunol.* **23,** 999–1028.

82. Weigert, M.G., Cesari, I.M., Yonkovich, S.J., and Cohn, M. (1970). Variability in the lambda light chain sequences of mouse antibody. *Nature* **228,** 1045–1047.

83. Borden, P., and Kabat, E.A. (1987). Nucleotide sequence of the cDNAs encoding the variable region heavy and light chains of a myeloma protein specific for the terminal nonreducing end of alpha(1–6)dextran. *Proc. Natl. Acad. Sci. USA* **84,** 2440–2443.

84. Hansburg, D., Perlmutter, R.M., Briles, D.E., and Davie, J.M. (1978). Analysis of the diversity of murine antibodies to dextran B1355. III. Idiotypic and spectrotypic correlations. *Eur. J. Immunol.* **8,** 352–359.

85. Kehry, M., Sibley, C., Fuhrman, J., Schilling, J., and Hood, L.E. (1979). Amino acid sequence of a mouse immunoglobulin mu chain. *Proc. Natl. Acad. Sci. USA* **76,** 2932–2936.

86. Hunkapiller, M.W., and Hood, L.E. (1978). Direct microsequence analysis of polypeptides using an improved sequenator, a nonprotein carrier (polybrene), and high pressure liquid chromatography. *Biochemistry* **17,** 2124–2133.

87. Sugii, S., Kabat, E.A., Shapiro, M., and Potter, M. (1981). Immunochemical specificity of the combining site of murine myeloma protein CAL20 TEPC1035 reactive with dextrans. *J. Exp. Med.* **153,** 166–181.

88. Shapiro, M., Personal Communication.

89. Takeo, K., and Kabat, E.A. (1978). Binding constants of dextrans and isomaltose oligosaccharides to dextran-specific myeloma proteins determined by affinity electrophoresis. *J. Immunol.* **121**, 2305–2310.

90. Padlan, E.A., and Kabat, E.A. (1988). Model-building study of the combining sites of two antibodies to alpha (1–6)dextran. *Proc. Natl. Acad. Sci. USA* **85**, 6885–6889.

91. Stein, K.E., Zopf, D.A., Miller, C.B., Johnson, B.M., Mongini, P.K., Ahmed, A., and Paul, W.E. (1983). Immune response to a thymus-dependent form of B512 dextran requires the presence of Lyb-5 + lymphocytes. *J. Exp. Med.* **157**, 657–666.

92. Matsuda, T., and Kabat, E.A. (1989). Variable region cDNA sequences and antigen binding specificity of mouse monoclonal antibodies to isomaltosyl oligosaccharides coupled to proteins. T-dependent analogues of alpha(1–6)dextran. *J. Immunol.* **142**, 863–870.

93. Blomberg, B., Geckeler, W.R., and Weigert, M. (1972). Genetics of the antibody response to dextran in mice. *Science* **177**, 178–180.

94. Newman, B.A., Liao, J., Gruezo, F., Sugii, S., Kabat, E.A., Torii, M., Clevinger, B.L., Davie, J.M., Schilling, J., Bond, M., and *et al.* (1986). Immunochemical studies of mouse monoclonal antibodies to dextran B1355S–II. Combining site specificity, sequence, idiotype and affinity. *Mol. Immunol.* **23**, 413–424.

95. Tittle, T.V., and Cohn, M. (1986). A characterization of the BALB/c lambda and kappa class antibodies to alpha (1,3) glycosidic linkages. *Cell Immunol.* **98**, 444–452.

96. Jennings, H.J. (1990). Capsular polysaccharides as vaccine candidates. *Curr. Top Microbiol. Immunol.* **150**, 97–127.

97. Robbins, J.B. (1978). Vaccines for the prevention of encapsulated bacterial diseases: current status, problems and prospects for the future. *Immunochemistry* **15**, 839–854.

98. Moxon, E.R., and Kroll, J.S. (1990). The role of bacterial polysaccharide capsules as virulence factors. *Curr. Top. Microbiol. Immunol.* **150**, 65–85.

99. Roberts, I.S. (1996). The biochemistry and genetics of capsular polysaccharide production in bacteria. *Annu. Rev. Microbiol.* **50**, 285–315.

100. Mandrell, R.E., and Zollinger, W.D. (1982). Measurement of antibodies to meningococcal group B polysaccharide: low avidity binding and equilibrium binding constants. *J. Immunol.* **129**, 2172–2178.

101. Avery, O., and Goebel, W. (1931). Chemo-immunological studies on conjugated carbohydrate-proteins. V. The immunological specificity of an antigen prepared by combining the capsular polysaccharide of type III pneumococcus with foreign protein. *J. Exp. Med.* **54**, 437–447.

102. Robbins, J.B., Parke, J.C., Jr., Schneerson, R., and Whisnant, J.K. (1973). Quantitative measurement of "natural" and immunization-induced *Haemophilus influenzae* type b capsular polysaccharide antibodies. *Pediatr. Res.* **7**, 103–110.

103. Crisel, R.M., Baker, R.S., and Dorman, D.E. (1975). Capsular polymer of *Haemophilus influenzae*, type b. I. Structural characterization of the capsular polymer of strain Eagan. *J. Biol. Chem.* **250**, 4926–4930.

104. Siber, G.R., Thompson, C., Reid, G.R., Almeido-Hill, J., Zacher, B., Wolff, M., and Santosham, M. (1992). Evaluation of bacterial polysaccharide immune globulin for the treatment or prevention of *Haemophilus influenzae* type b and pneumococcal disease. *J. Infect. Dis. 165 Suppl.* **1**, S129–133.

105. Tarrand, J.J., Scott, M.G., Takes, P.A., and Nahm, M.H. (1989). Clonal characterization of the human IgG antibody repertoire to *Haemophilus influenzae* type B polysaccharide. Demonstration of three types of V regions and their association with H and L chain isotypes. *J. Immunol.* **142**, 2519–2526.

106. Schneerson, R., Rodrigues, L.P., Parke, J.C., Jr., and Robbins, J.B. (1971). Immunity to disease caused by Hemophilus influenzae type b. II. Specificity and some biologic

characteristics of "natural," infection-acquired, and immunization-induced antibodies to the capsular polysaccharide of *Hemophilus influenzae* type b. *J. Immunol.* **107,** 1081–1089.

107. Chung, G.H., Scott, M.G., Kim, K.H., Kearney, J., Siber, G.R., Ambrosino, D.M., and Nahm, M.H. (1993). Clonal characterization of the human IgG antibody repertoire to *Haemophilus influenzae* type b polysaccharide. V. *In vivo* expression of individual antibody clones is dependent on Ig CH haplotypes and the categories of antigen. *J. Immunol.* **151,** 4352–4361.

108. Insel, R.A., and Anderson, P.W. (1986). Oligosaccharide-protein conjugate vaccines induce and prime for oligoclonal IgG antibody responses to the *Haemophilus influenzae* b capsular polysaccharide in human infants. *J. Exp. Med.* **163,** 262–269.

109. Nahm, M.H., Kim, K.H., Anderson, P., Hetherington, S.V., and Park, M.K. (1995). Functional capacities of clonal antibodies to *Haemophilus influenzae* type b polysaccharide. *Infect. Immun.* **63,** 2989–2994.

110. Barington, T., Hougs, L., Juul, L., Madsen, H.O., Ryder, L.P., Heilmann, C., and Svejgaard, A. (1996). The progeny of a single virgin B cell predominates the human recall B cell response to the capsular polysaccharide of *Haemophilus influenzae* type b. *J. Immunol.* **157,** 4016–4027.

111. Silverman, G.J., and Lucas, A.H. (1991). Variable region diversity in human circulating antibodies specific for the capsular polysaccharide of *Haemophilus influenzae* type b. Preferential usage of two types of VH3 heavy chains. *J. Clin. Invest.* **88,** 911–920.

112. Scott, M.G., and Nahm, M.H. (1992). Characterization of the human IgG antibody VL repertoire to *Haemophilus influenzae* type b polysaccharide. *J. Infect. Dis.* 165 Suppl. **1,** S53–56.

113. Adderson, E.E., Shackelford, P.G., Quinn, A., and Carroll, W.L. (1991). Restricted Ig H chain V gene usage in the human antibody response to *Haemophilus influenzae* type b capsular polysaccharide. *J. Immunol.* **147,** 1667–1674.

114. Adderson, E.E., Shackelford, P.G., Quinn, A., Wilson, P.M., Cunningham, M.W., Insel, R.A., and Carroll, W.L. (1993). Restricted immunoglobulin VH usage and VDJ combinations in the human response to *Haemophilus influenzae* type b capsular polysaccharide. Nucleotide sequences of monospecific anti-Haemophilus antibodies and polyspecific antibodies cross-reacting with self antigens. *J. Clin. Invest.* **91,** 2734–2743.

115. Lucas, A.H., and Granoff, D.M. (1990). A major crossreactive idiotype associated with human antibodies to the *Haemophilus influenzae* b polysaccharide. Expression in relation to age and immunoglobulin G subclass. *J. Clin. Invest.* **85,** 1158–1166.

116. Lucas, A.H., Langley, R.J., Granoff, D.M., Nahm, M.H., Kitamura, M.Y., and Scott, M.G. (1991). An idiotypic marker associated with a germ-line encoded kappa light chain variable region that predominates the vaccine-induced human antibody response to the *Haemophilus influenzae* b polysaccharide. *J. Clin. Invest.* **88,** 1811–1818.

117. Scott, M.G., Crimmins, D.L., McCourt, D.W., Zocher, I., Thiebe, R., Zachau, H.G., and Nahm, M.H. (1989). Clonal characterization of the human IgG antibody repertoire to *Haemophilus influenzae* type b polysaccharide. III. A single VKII gene and one of several JK genes are joined by an invariant arginine to form the most common L chain V region. *J. Immunol.* **143,** 4110–4116.

118. Scott, M.G., Crimmins, D.L., McCourt, D.W., Chung, G., Schable, K.F., Thiebe, R., Quenzel, E.M., Zachau, H.G., and Nahm, M.H. (1991). Clonal characterization of the human IgG antibody repertoire to *Haemophilus influenzae* type b polysaccharide. IV. The less frequently expressed VL are heterogeneous. *J. Immunol.* **147,** 4007–4013.

119. Adderson, E.E., Shackelford, P.G., Insel, R.A., Quinn, A., Wilson, P.M., and Carroll, W.L. (1992). Immunoglobulin light chain variable region gene sequences for human antibodies to *Haemophilus influenzae* type b capsular polysaccharide are dominated by

a limited number of V kappa and V lambda segments and VJ combinations. *J. Clin. Invest.* **89**, 729–738.

120. Lucas, A.H., Larrick, J.W., and Reason, D.C. (1994). Variable region sequences of a protective human monoclonal antibody specific for the *Haemophilus influenzae* type b capsular polysaccharide. *Infect Immun.* **62**, 3873–3880.

121. Scott, M.G., Tarrand, J.J., Crimmins, D.L., McCourt, D.W., Siegel, N.R., Smith, C.E., and Nahm, M.H. (1989). Clonal characterization of the human IgG antibody repertoire to *Haemophilus influenzae* type b polysaccharide. II. IgG antibodies contain VH genes from a single VH family and VL genes from at least four VL families. *J. Immunol.* **143**, 293–298.

122. Feeney, A.J., Atkinson, M.J., Cowan, M.J., Escuro, G., and Lugo, G. (1996). A defective Vkappa A2 allele in Navajos which may play a role in susceptibility to *Haemophilus influenzae* type b disease. *J. Clin. Invest.* **97**, 2277–2282.

123. Granoff, D.M., and Lucas, A.H. (1995). Laboratory correlates of protection against *Haemophilus influenzae* type b disease. Importance of assessment of antibody avidity and immunologic memory. *Ann. N Y Acad. Sci.* **754**, 278–288.

124. Lucas, A.H., and Granoff, D.M. (1995). Functional differences in idiotypically defined IgG1 anti-polysaccharide antibodies elicited by vaccination with *Haemophilus influenzae* type B polysaccharide-protein conjugates. *J. Immunol.* **154**, 4195–4202.

125. Evans, A., and Brachman, P. (1998). *Bacterial infections of humans, epidemiology and control.* Kluwer Academic/Plenum Publishers, New York.

126. Le Moli, S., Matricardi, P.M., Quinti, I., Stroffolini, T., and D'Amelio, R. (1991). Clonotypic analysis of human antibodies specific for *Neisseria meningitidis* polysaccharides A and C in adults. *Clin. Exp. Immunol.* **83**, 460–465.

127. Gold, R., Lepow, M.L., Goldschneider, I., Draper, T.F., and Gotschlich, E.C. (1978). Antibody responses of human infants to three doses of group A *Neisseria meningitidis* polysaccharide vaccine administered at two, four, and six months of age. *J. Infect. Dis.* **138**, 731–735.

128. Wilkins, J., and Wehrle, P.F. (1979). Further characterization of responses of infants and children to meningococcal A polysaccharide vaccine. *J. Pediatr.* **94**, 828–832.

129. Kayhty, H., Karanko, V., Peltola, H., Sarna, S., and Makela, P.H. (1980). Serum antibodies to capsular polysaccharide vaccine of group A *Neissera meningitidis* followed for three years in infants and children. *J. Infect. Dis.* **142**, 861–868.

130. Muller, E., and Apicella, M.A. (1988). T-cell modulation of the murine antibody response to *Neisseria meningitidis* group A capsular polysaccharide. *Infect. Immun.* **56**, 259–266.

131. Liu, T.Y., Gotschlich, E.C., Dunne, F.T., and Jonssen, E.K. (1971). Studies on the meningococcal polysaccharides. II. Composition and chemical properties of the group B and group C polysaccharide. *J. Biol. Chem.* **246**, 4703–4712.

132. Finne, J., Leinonen, M., and Makela, P.H. (1983). Antigenic similarities between brain components and bacteria causing meningitis. Implications for vaccine development and pathogenesis. *Lancet* **2**, 355–357.

133. Colino, J., and Outschoorn, I. (1998). Dynamics of the murine humoral immune response to *Neisseria meningitis* group B capsular polysaccharide. *Infect. Immun.* **66**, 505–513.

134. Frosch, M., Gorgen, I., Boulnois, G.J., Timmis, K.N., and Bitter-Suermann, D. (1985). NZB mouse system for production of monoclonal antibodies to weak bacterial antigens: isolation of an IgG antibody to the polysaccharide capsules of *Escherichia coli* K1 and group B meningococci. *Proc. Natl. Acad. Sci. USA* **82**, 1194–1198.

135. Vaesen, M., Frosch, M., Weisgerber, C., Eckart, K., Kratzin, H., Bitter-Suermann, D., and Hilschmann, N. (1991). Primary structure of the murine monoclonal IgG2a antibody mAb735 against alpha(2–8) polysialic acid. 1) Amino-acid sequence of the light (L-) chain, kappa-isotype. *Biol. Chem. Hoppe Seyler* **372**, 451–453.

136. Klebert, S., Kratzin, H.D., Zimmermann, B., Vaesen, M., Frosch, M., Weisgerber, C., Bitter-Suermann, D., and Hilschmann, N. (1993). Primary structure of the murine monoclonal IgG2a antibody mAb735 against alpha (2–8) polysialic acid. 2. Amino acid sequence of the heavy (H-) chain Fd' region. *Biol. Chem. Hoppe Seyler* **374,** 993–1000.

137. Pon, R.A., Lussier, M., Yang, Q.L., and Jennings, H.J. (1997). N-Propionylated group B meningococcal polysaccharide mimics a unique bactericidal capsular epitope in group B *Neisseria meningitidis. J. Exp. Med.* **185,** 1929–1938.

138. Lifely, M.R., and Esdaile, J. (1991). Specificity of the immune response to the group B polysaccharide of *Neisseria meningitidis. Immunology* **74,** 490–496.

139. Granoff, D.M., Bartoloni, A., Ricci, S., Gallo, E., Rosa, D., Ravenscroft, N., Guarnieri, V., Seid, R.C., Shan, A., Usinger, W.R., Tan, S., McHugh, Y.E., and Moe, G.R. (1998). Bactericidal monoclonal antibodies that define unique meningococcal B polysaccharide epitopes that do not cross-react with human polysialic acid. *J. Immunol.* **160,** 5028–5036.

140. Devi, S.J., Karpas, A.B., and Frasch, C.E. (1996). Binding diversity of monoclonal antibodies to alpha(2->8) polysialic acid conjugated to outer membrane vesicle via adipic acid dihydrazide. *FEMS Immunol. Med. Microbiol.* **14,** 211–220.

141. Raff, H.V., Devereux, D., Shuford, W., Abbott-Brown, D., and Maloney, G. (1988). Human monoclonal antibody with protective activity for *Escherichia coli* K1 and *Neisseria meningitidis* group B infections. *J. Infect. Dis.* **157,** 118–126.

142. Azmi, F.H., Lucas, A.H., Raff, H.V., and Granoff, D.M. (1994). Variable region sequences and idiotypic expression of a protective human immunoglobulin M antibody to capsular polysaccharides of *Neisseria meningitidis* group B and *Escherichia coli* K1. *Infect. Immun.* **62,** 1776–1786.

143. Kabat, E.A., Nickerson, K.G., Liao, J., Grossbard, L., Osserman, E.F., Glickman, E., Chess, L., Robbins, J.B., Schneerson, R., and Yang, Y.H. (1986). A human monoclonal macroglobulin with specificity for alpha(2–8)-linked poly-N-acetyl neuraminic acid, the capsular polysaccharide of group B meningococci and *Escherichia coli* K1, which crossreacts with polynucleotides and with denatured DNA. *J. Exp. Med.* **164,** 642–654.

144. Gawinowicz, M.A., Merlini, G., Birken, S., Osserman, E.F., and Kabat, E.A. (1991). Amino acid sequence of the FV region of a human monoclonal IgM (NOV) with specificity for the capsular polysaccharide of the group B meningococcus and of *Escherichia coli* K1, which cross-reacts with polynucleotides and with denatured DNA. *J. Immunol.* **147,** 915–920.

145. Azmi, F.H., Lucas, A.H., Spiegelberg, H.L., and Granoff, D.M. (1995). Human immunoglobulin M paraproteins cross-reactive with *Neisseria meningitidis* group B polysaccharide and fetal brain. *Infect. Immun.* **63,** 1906–1913.

146. Bhattacharjee, A.K., Jennings, H.J., Kenny, C.P., Martin, A., and Smith, I.C.P. (1975). Structural determination of the sialic acid polysaccharide antigens of *Neisseria meningitidis* serogroups B and C with carbon 13 nuclear magnetic resonance. *J. Biol. Chem.* **250,** 1926–1932.

147. Rubinstein, L.J., Garcia-Ojeda, P.A., Michon, F., Jennings, H.J., and Stein, K.E. (1998). Murine immune responses to *Neisseria meningitidis* group C capsular polysaccharide and a thymus-dependent toxoid conjugate vaccine. *Infect. Immun.* **66,** 5450–5456.

148. Rubinstein, L.J., and Stein, K.E. (1988). Murine immune response to the *Neisseria meningitidis* group C capsular polysaccharide. I., Ontogeny. *J. Immunol.* **141,** 4352–4356.

149. Goldschneider, I., Gotschlich, E.C., and Artenstein, M.S. (1969). Human immunity to the meningococcus. I. The role of humoral antibodies. *J. Exp. Med.* **129,** 1307–1326.

150. Rubinstein, L.J., and Stein, K.E. (1988). Murine immune response to the *Neisseria meningitidis* group C capsular polysaccharide. II. Specificity. *J. Immunol.* **141,** 4357–4362.

151. Garcia-Ojeda, P. Unpublished data.

152. Smithson, S.L., Srivastava, N., Hutchins, W.A., and Westerink, M.A. (1999). Molecular analysis of the heavy chain of antibodies that recognize the capsular polysaccharide of *Neisseria meningitidis* in hu-PBMC reconstituted SCID mice and in the immunized human donor. *Mol. Immunol.* **36**, 113–124.

153. Lancefield, R. (1933). A serological differentiation of human and other groups of hemolytic streptococci. *J. Exp. Med.* **57**, 571–595.

154. Fulton, R.J., and Davie, J.M. (1984). Influence of the immunoglobulin heavy chain locus on expression of the VK1GAC light chain. *J. Immunol.* **133**, 465–470.

155. Nahm, M.H., Clevinger, B.L., and Davie, J.M. (1982). Monoclonal antibodies to streptococcal group A carbohydrate. I. A dominant idiotypic determinant is located on Vk. *J. Immunol.* **129**, 1513–1518.

156. Chang, J.Y., Herbst, H., Aebersold, R., and Braun, D.G. (1983). A new isotype sequence (V kappa 27) of the variable region of kappa-light chains from a mouse hybridoma-derived anti-(streptococcal group A polysaccharide) antibody containing an additional cysteine residue. Application of the dimethylaminoazobenzene isothiocyanate technique for the isolation of peptides. *Biochem. J.* **211**, 173–180.

157. Lutz, C.T., Bartholow, T.L., Greenspan, N.S., Fulton, R.J., Monafo, W.J., Perlmutter, R.M., Huang, H.V., and Davie, J.M. (1987). Molecular dissection of the murine antibody response to streptococcal group A carbohydrate. *J. Exp. Med.* **165**, 531–545.

158. Phillips, N.J., and Davie, J.M. (1990). Idiotope structure and genetic diversity in antistreptococcal group A carbohydrate antibodies. *J. Immunol.* **145**, 915–924.

159. Jarvis, C.D., Cannon, L.E., and Stavnezer, J. (1989). Mouse antibody response to group A streptococcal carbohydrate. *J. Immunol.* **143**, 4213–4220.

160. Shackelford, P.G., Nelson, S.J., Palma, A.T., and Nahm, M.H. (1988). Human antibodies to group A streptococcal carbohydrate. Ontogeny, subclass restriction, and clonal diversity. *J. Immunol.* **140**, 3200–3205.

161. Wilkinson, H.W., Facklam, R.R., and Wortham, E.C. (1973). Distribution by serological type of group B streptococci isolated from a variety of clinical material over a five-year period (with special reference to neonatal sepsis and meningitis). *Infect. Immun.* **8**, 228–235.

162. Baker, C.J., and Barrett, F.F. (1973). Transmission of group B streptococci among parturient women and their neonates. *J. Pediatr.* **83**, 919–925.

163. Baker, C.J., Edwards, M.S., and Kasper, D.L. (1981). Role of antibody to native type III polysaccharide of group B *Streptococcus* in infant infection. *Pediatrics* **68**, 544–549.

164. Paoletti, L.C., Wessels, M.R., Michon, F., DiFabio, J., Jennings, H.J., and Kasper, D.L. (1992). Group B Streptococcus type II polysaccharide-tetanus toxoid conjugate vaccine. *Infect. Immun.* **60**, 4009–4014.

165. Baker, C.J., Paoletti, L.C., Wessels, M.R., Guttormsen, H.K., Rench, M.A., Hickman, M.E., and Kasper, D.L. (1999). Safety and immunogenicity of capsular polysaccharide-tetanus toxoid conjugate vaccines for group B streptococcal types Ia and Ib. *J. Infect. Dis.* **179**, 142–150.

166. Kasper, D.L., Paoletti, L.C., Wessels, M.R., Guttormsen, H.K., Carey, V.J., Jennings, H.J., and Baker, C.J. (1996). Immune response to type III group B streptococcal polysaccharide-tetanus toxoid conjugate vaccine. *J. Clin. Invest.* **98**, 2308–2314.

167. Wessels, M.R., Paoletti, L.C., Pinel, J., and Kasper, D.L. (1995). Immunogenicity and protective activity in animals of a type V group B streptococcal polysaccharide-tetanus toxoid conjugate vaccine. *J. Infect. Dis.* **171**, 879–884.

168. Egan, M.L., Pritchard, D.G., Dillon, H.C., Jr., and Gray, B.M. (1983). Protection of mice from experimental infection with type III group B Streptococcus using monoclonal antibodies. *J. Exp. Med.* **158**, 1006–1011.

169. Raff, H.V., Siscoe, P.J., Wolff, E.A., Maloney, G., and Shuford, W. (1988). Human monoclonal antibodies to group B streptococcus. Reactivity and *in vivo* protection against multiple serotypes. *J. Exp. Med.* **168**, 905–917.

170. Feldman, R.G., Breukels, M.A., David, S., and Rijkers, G.T. (1998). Properties of human anti-group B streptococcal type III capsular IgG antibody. *Clin. Immunol. Immunopathol.* **86,** 161–169.

171. Zou, W., Mackenzie, R., Therien, L., Hirama, T., Yang, Q., Gidney, M.A., and Jennings, H.J. (1999). Conformational epitope of the type III group B *Streptococcus* capsular polysaccharide. *J. Immunol.* **163,** 820–825.

172. Butler, J.C., Dowell, S.F., and Breiman, R.F. (1998). Epidemiology of emerging pneumococcal drug resistance: implications for treatment and prevention. *Vaccine* **16,** 1693–1697.

173. Black, S., Shinefield, H., Fireman, B., Lewis, E., Ray, P., Hansen, J.R., Elvin, L., Ensor, K.M., Hackell, J., Siber, G., Malinoski, F., Madore, D., Chang, I., Kohberger, R., Watson, W., Austrian, R., and Edwards, K. (2000). Efficacy, safety and immunogenicity of heptavalent pneumococcal conjugate vaccine in children. Northern California Kaiser Permanente Vaccine Study Center Group. *Pediatr.* **19,** 187–195.

174. Brundish, D., and Baddiley, J. (1968). Pneumococcal C-substance, a ribitol teichoic acid containing choline phosphate. *Biochem. J.* **110,** 573–582.

175. Briles, D.E., Nahm, M., Schroer, K., Davie, J., Baker, P., Kearney, J., and Barletta, R. (1981). Antiphosphocholine antibodies found in normal mouse serum are protective against intravenous infection with type 3 *Streptococcus pneumoniae*. *J. Exp. Med.* **153,** 694–705.

176. Wallick, S., Claflin, J.L., and Briles, D.E. (1983). Resistance to *Streptococcus pneumoniae* is induced by a phosphocholine-protein conjugate. *J. Immunol.* **130,** 2871–2875.

177. Musher, D.M., Watson, D.A., and Baughn, R.E. (1990). Does naturally acquired IgG antibody to cell wall polysaccharide protect human subjects against pneumococcal infection? *J. Infect. Dis.* **161,** 736–740.

178. Nielsen, S.V., Sorensen, U.B., and Henrichsen, J. (1993). Antibodies against pneumococcal C-polysaccharide are not protective. *Microb. Pathog.* **14,** 299–305.

179. Skov Sorensen, U.B., Blom, J., Birch-Andersen, A., and Henrichsen, J. (1988). Ultrastructural localization of capsules, cell wall polysaccharide, cell wall proteins, and F antigen in pneumococci. *Infect. Immun.* **56,** 1890–1896.

180. Kolberg, J., Aaberge, I.S., Jantzen, E., Lovik, M., Lermark, G., and Steen, T. (1992). Murine monoclonal antibodies against pneumococcal capsular polysaccharide types 4, 8, 22F and 19A/19F. *Apmis* **100,** 91–94.

181. Kolberg, J., and Jones, C. (1998). Monoclonal antibodies with specificities for *Streptococcus pneumoniae* group 9 capsular polysaccharides. *FEMS Immunol. Med. Microbiol.* **20,** 249–255.

182. Lu, C., Lee, C., and Kind, P. (1994). Immune responses of young mice to pneumococcal type 9V polysaccharide-tetanus toxoid conjugate. *Infect. Immun.* **62,** 2754–2760.

183. Lucas, A.H., Granoff, D.M., Mandrell, R.E., Connolly, C.C., Shan, A.S., and Powers, D.C. (1997). Oligoclonality of serum immunoglobulin G antibody responses to *Streptococcus pneumoniae* capsular polysaccharide serotypes 6B, 14, and 23F. *Infect. Immun.* **65,** 5103–5109.

184. Park, M.K., Sun, Y., Olander, J.V., Hoffmann, J.W., and Nahm, M.H. (1996). The repertoire of human antibodies to the carbohydrate capsule of *Streptococcus pneumoniae* 6B. *J. Infect. Dis.* **174,** 75–82.

185. Baxendale, H.E., Davis, Z., White, H.N., Spellerberg, M.B., Stevenson, F.K., and Goldblatt, D. (2000). Immunogenetic analysis of the immune response to pneumococcal polysaccharide. *Eur. J. Immunol.* **30,** 1214–1223.

186. Sun, Y., Park, M.K., Kim, J., Diamond, B., Solomon, A., and Nahm, M.H. (1999). Repertoire of human antibodies against the polysaccharide capsule of *Streptococcus pneumoniae* serotype 6B. *Infect. Immun.* **67,** 1172–1179.

187. Usinger, W.R., and Lucas, A.H. (1999). Avidity as a determinant of the protective efficacy of human antibodies to pneumococcal capsular polysaccharides. *Infect. Immun.* **67,** 2366–2370.

188. Soininen, A., Seppala, I., Nieminen, T., Eskola, J., and Kayhty, H. (1999). IgG subclass distribution of antibodies after vaccination of adults with pneumococcal conjugate vaccines. *Vaccine* **17,** 1889–1897.
189. Barrett, D.J., Lee, C.G., Ammann, A.J., and Ayoub, E.M. (1984). IgG and IgM pneumococcal polysaccharide antibody responses in infants. *Pediatr. Res.* **18,** 1067–1071.
190. Lawrence, E.M., Edwards, K.M., Schiffman, G., Thompson, J.M., Vaughn, W.K., and Wright, P.F. (1983). Pneumococcal vaccine in normal children. Primary and secondary vaccination. *Am. J. Dis. Child.* **137,** 846–850.
191. Ahman, H., Kayhty, H., Tamminen, P., Vuorela, A., Malinoski, F., and Eskola, J. (1996). Pentavalent pneumococcal oligosaccharide conjugate vaccine PncCRM is well-tolerated and able to induce an antibody response in infants. Pediatr. Infect. Dis. J. **15,** 134–139.
192. Vidarsson, G., Sigurdardottir, S.T., Gudnason, T., Kjartansson, S., Kristinsson, K.G., Ingolfsdottir, G., Jonsson, S., Valdimarsson, H., Schiffman, G., Schneerson, R., and Jonsdottir, I. (1998). Isotypes and opsonophagocytosis of pneumococcus type 6B antibodies elicited in infants and adults by an experimental pneumococcus type 6B-tetanus toxoid vaccine. Infect. Immun. **66,** 2866–2870.
193. Anttila, M., Eskola, J., Ahman, H., and Kayhty, H. (1998). Avidity of IgG for *Streptococcus pneumoniae* type 6B and 23F polysaccharides in infants primed with pneumococcal conjugates and boosted with polysaccharide or conjugate vaccines. *J. Infect. Dis.* **177,** 1614–1621.
194. Daum, R.S., Hogerman, D., Rennels, M.B., Bewley, K., Malinoski, F., Rothstein, E., Reisinger, K., Block, S., Keyserling, H., and Steinhoff, M. (1997). Infant immunization with pneumococcal CRM197 vaccines: effect of saccharide size on immunogenicity and interactions with simultaneously administered vaccines. *J. Infect. Dis.* **176,** 445–455.
195. Anttila, M., Eskola, J., Ahman, H., and Kayhty, H. (1999). Differences in the avidity of antibodies evoked by four different pneumococcal conjugate vaccines in early childhood. *Vaccine* **17,** 1970–1977.
196. Kaplan, J.E., Jones, J.L., and Dykewicz, C.A. (2000). Protists as opportunistic pathogens: public health impact in the 1990s and beyond. *J. Eukaryot Microbiol.* **47,** 15–20.
197. Cherniak, R., and Sundstrom, J.B. (1994). Polysaccharide antigens of the capsule of *Cryptococcus neoformans*. *Infect. Immun.* **62,** 1507–1512.
198. Casadevall, A., and Scharff, M.D. (1991). The mouse antibody response to infection with *Cryptococcus neoformans*: VH and VL usage in polysaccharide binding antibodies. *J. Exp. Med.* **174,** 151–160.
199. Mukherjee, J., Casadevall, A., and Scharff, M.D. (1993). Molecular characterization of the humoral responses to *Cryptococcus neoformans* infection and glucuronoxylomannan-tetanus toxoid conjugate immunization. *J. Exp. Med.* **177,** 1105–1116.
200. Nussbaum, G., Anandasabapathy, S., Mukherjee, J., Fan, M., Casadevall, A., and Scharff, M.D. (1999). Molecular and idiotypic analyses of the antibody response to *Cryptococcus neoformans* glucuronoxylomannan-protein conjugate vaccine in autoimmune and nonautoimmune mice. *Infect. Immun.* **67,** 4469–4476.
201. Casadevall, A., DeShaw, M., Fan, M., Dromer, F., Kozel, T.R., and Pirofski, L.A. (1994). Molecular and idiotypic analysis of antibodies to *Cryptococcus neoformans* glucuronoxylomannan. *Infect. Immun.* **62,** 3864–3872.
202. Belay, T., Cherniak, R., Kozel, T.R., and Casadevall, A. (1997). Reactivity patterns and epitope specificities of anti-*Cryptococcus neoformans* monoclonal antibodies by enzyme-linked immunosorbent assay and dot enzyme assay. *Infect. Immun.* **65,** 718–728.
203. Pirofski, L., Lui, R., DeShaw, M., Kressel, A.B., and Zhong, Z. (1995). Analysis of human monoclonal antibodies elicited by vaccination with a *Cryptococcus*

neoformans glucuronoxylomannan capsular polysaccharide vaccine. *Infect. Immun.* **63,** 3005–3014.

204. Achi, R., Dac Cam, P., Forsum, U., Karlsson, K., Saenz, P., Mata, L., and Lindberg, A.A. (1992). Titres of class-specific antibodies against Shigella and Salmonella lipopolysaccharide antigens in colostrum and breast milk of Costa Rican, Swedish and Vietnamese mothers. *J. Infect.* **25,** 89–105.

205. Law, D. (2000). Virulence factors of *Escherichia coli* O157 and other Shiga toxin-producing E. coli. *J. Appl. Microbiol.* **88,** 729–745.

206. Stroeher, U.H., Jedani, K.E., and Manning, P.A. (1998). Genetic organization of the regions associated with surface polysaccharide synthesis in *Vibrio cholerae* O1, O139 and *Vibrio anguillarum* O1 and O2: a review. *Gene* **223,** 269–282.

207. Heyns, K., Kiessling, G., Lindenberg, W., Paulsen, H., and Webster, M. (1959). D-galaktosaminuronsaure (2-amino-2deoxy-D-galakturonsaure) als baustein des Vi-antigens. *Chem. Ber.* **92,** 2435–2437.

208. Tsang, R.S., and Chau, P.Y. (1987). Production of Vi monoclonal antibodies and their application as diagnostic reagents. *J. Clin. Microbiol.* **25,** 531–535.

209. Luk, J.M., Zhao, C.R., Karlsson, K.M., and Lindberg, A.A. (1992). Specificity of monoclonal antibodies binding to the polysaccharide antigens (Vi, O9) of *Salmonella typhi*. *FEMS Microbiol. Lett.* **76,** 173–178.

210. Pienkowska, D., Kunikowska, D., and Glosnicka, R. (1993). Monoclonal antibodies against Vi antigen production and characterization. *Bull. Inst. Mar. Trop. Med. Gdynia* **44,** 89–93.

211. Kossaczka, Z., Lin, F.Y., Ho, V.A., Thuy, N.T., Van Bay, P., Thanh, T.C., Khiem, H.B., Trach, D.D., Karpas, A., Hunt, S., Bryla, D.A., Schneerson, R., Robbins, J.B., and Szu, S.C. (1999). Safety and immunogenicity of Vi conjugate vaccines for typhoid fever in adults, teenagers, and 2- to 4-year-old children in Vietnam. *Infect. Immun.* **67,** 5806–5810.

212. Pier, G.B., Matthews, W.J., Jr., and Eardley, D.D. (1983). Immunochemical characterization of the mucoid exopolysaccharide of *Pseudomonas aeruginosa*. *J. Infect. Dis.* **147,** 494–503.

213. Pier, G.B., Small, G.J., and Warren, H.B. (1990). Protection against mucoid *Pseudomonas aeruginosa* in rodent models of endobronchial infections. *Science* **249,** 537–540.

214. Pier, G.B., Saunders, J.M., Ames, P., Edwards, M.S., Auerbach, H., Goldfarb, J., Speert, D.P., and Hurwitch, S. (1987). Opsonophagocytic killing antibody to *Pseudomonas aeruginosa* mucoid exopolysaccharide in older noncolonized patients with cystic fibrosis. *N. Engl. J. Med.* **317,** 793–798.

215. Tosi, M.F., Zakem-Cloud, H., Demko, C.A., Schreiber, J.R., Stern, R.C., Konstan, M.W., and Berger, M. (1995). Cross-sectional and longitudinal studies of naturally occurring antibodies to *Pseudomonas aeruginosa* in cystic fibrosis indicate absence of antibody-mediated protection and decline in opsonic quality after infection. *J. Infect. Dis.* **172,** 453–461.

216. Devi, S.J., Robbins, J.B., and Schneerson, R. (1991). Antibodies to poly[(2–8)-alpha-N-acetylneuraminic acid] and poly[(2–9)-alpha-N-acetylneuraminic acid] are elicited by immunization of mice with *Escherichia coli* K92 conjugates: potential vaccines for groups B and C meningococci and *E. coli* K1. *Proc. Natl. Acad. Sci. USA* **88,** 7175–7179.

217. Kaijser, B., and Ahlstedt, S. (1977). Protective capacity of antibodies against *Escherichia coli* and K antigens. *Infect. Immun.* **17,** 286–289.

218. Kim, K.S., Kang, J.H., Cross, A.S., Kaufman, B., Zollinger, W., and Sadoff, J. (1988). Functional activities of monoclonal antibodies to the O side chain of *Escherichia coli* lipopolysaccharides *in vitro* and *in vivo*. *J. Infect. Dis.* **157,** 47–53.

219. Orskov, I., and Orskov, F. (1984). Serotyping of Klebsiella. *Methods Microbiol.* **14,** 143–164.

220. Lang, A.B., Bruderer, U., Senyk, G., Pitt, T.L., Larrick, J.W., and Cryz, S.J., Jr. (1991). Human monoclonal antibodies specific for capsular polysaccharides of Klebsiella recognize clusters of multiple serotypes. *J. Immunol.* **146,** 3160–3164.

221. Trautmann, M., Cryz, S.J., Jr., Sadoff, J.C., and Cross, A.S. (1988). A murine monoclonal antibody against Klebsiella capsular polysaccharide is opsonic *in vitro* and protects against experimental *Klebsiella pneumoniae* infection. *Microb. Pathog.* **5,** 177–187.

222. Held, T.K., Trautmann, M., Mielke, M.E., Neudeck, H., Cryz, S.J., Jr., and Cross, A.S. (1992). Monoclonal antibody against Klebsiella capsular polysaccharide reduces severity and hematogenic spread of experimental *Klebsiella pneumoniae* pneumonia. *Infect. Immun.* **60,** 1771–1778.

223. Rukavina, T., Ticac, B., Susa, M., Jendrike, N., Jonjic, S., Lucin, P., Marre, R., Doric, M., and Trautmann, M. (1997). Protective effect of antilipopolysaccharide monoclonal antibody in experimental Klebsiella infection. *Infect. Immun.* **65,** 1754–1760.

224. Held, T.K., Jendrike, N.R., Rukavina, T., Podschun, R., and Trautmann, M. (2000). Binding to and opsonophagocytic activity of O-antigen-specific monoclonal antibodies against encapsulated and nonencapsulated *Klebsiella pneumoniae* serotype O1 strains. *Infect. Immun.* **68,** 2402–2409.

225. Thurin, J. (1988). Binding sites of monoclonal anti-carbohydrate antibodies. *Curr. Top Microbiol. Immunol.* **139,** 59–79.

226. Kimura, H., Umeda, M., and Marcus, D.M. (1989). Expression of a cross-reactive idiotope on naturally occurring murine antibodies against 3-fucosyllactosamine, levan, and dextran. *J. Immunol.* **142,** 3477–3481.

227. Dinh, Q., Weng, N.P., Kiso, M., Ishida, H., Hasegawa, A., and Marcus, D.M. (1996). High affinity antibodies against Lex and sialyl Lex from a phage display library. *J. Immunol.* **157,** 732–738.

228. Marcus, D.M., Perry, L., Gilbert, S., Preud'homme, J.L., and Kyle, R. (1989). Human IgM monoclonal proteins that bind 3-fucosyllactosamine, asialo-GM1, and GM1. *J. Immunol.* **143,** 2929–2932.

229. Cerato, E., Birkle, S., Portoukalian, J., Mezazigh, A., Chatal, J.F., and Aubry, J. (1997). Variable region gene segments of nine monoclonal antibodies specific to disialogangliosides (GD2, GD3) and their O-acetylated derivatives. *Hybridoma* **16,** 307–316.

230. Zenita, K., Hirashima, K., Shigeta, K., Hiraiwa, N., Takada, A., Hashimoto, K., Fujimoto, E., Yago, K., and Kannagi, R. (1990). Northern hybridization analysis of VH gene expression in murine monoclonal antibodies directed to cancer-associated ganglioside antigens having various sialic acid linkages. *J. Immunol.* **144,** 4442–4451.

231. Snyder, J.G., Weng, N., Yu-Lee, L.Y., and Marcus, D.M. (1990). Heavy and light chain sequences of four monoclonal antibodies that bind galactosylgloboside (GalGb4). *Eur. J. Immunol.* **20,** 2673–2677.

232. Snyder, J.G., Dinh, Q., Morrison, S.L., Padlan, E.A., Mitchell, M., Yu-Lee, L.Y., and Marcus, D.M. (1994). Structure-function studies of anti-3-fucosyllactosamine (Le(x)) and galactosylgloboside antibodies. *J. Immunol.* **153,** 1161–1170.

233. Nishinaka, Y., Hoon, D.S.B., and Irie, R.F. (1998). Human IgM antibodies to tumor-associated gangliosides share VHIII (V3–23) and VKIV family subgroups. *Immunogenetics* **48,** 73–75.

234. Mukerjee, S., Nasoff, M., McKnight, M., and Glassy, M. (1998). Characterization of human IgG1 monoclonal antibody against gangliosides expressed on tumor cells. *Hybridoma* **17,** 133–142.

235. Silverman, G.J., and Carson, D.A. (1990). Structural characterization of human monoclonal cold agglutinins: evidence for a distinct primary sequence-defined VH4 idiotype. *Eur. J. Immunol.* **20,** 351–356.

236. Silberstein, L.E., Jefferies, L.C., Goldman, J., Friedman, D., Moore, J.S., Nowell, P.C., Roelcke, D., Pruzanski, W., Roudier, J., and Silverman, G.J. (1991). Variable region

gene analysis of pathologic human autoantibodies to the related i and I red blood cell antigens. *Blood* **78**, 2372–2386.

237. Li, Y., Spellerberg, M.B., Stevenson, F.K., Capra, J.D., and Potter, K.N. (1996). The I binding specificity of human VH 4–34 (VH 4–21) encoded antibodies is determined by both VH framework region 1 and complementarity determining region 3. *J. Mol. Biol.* **256**, 577–589.

238. Dall'Acqua, W., Goldman, E.R., Lin, W., Teng, C., Tsuchiya, D., Li, H., Ysern, X., Braden, B.C., Li, Y., Smith-Gill, S.J., and Mariuzza, R.A. (1998). A mutational analysis of binding interactions in an antigen-antibody protein-protein complex. *Biochemistry* **37**, 7981–7991.

239. Brady, R.L., Edwards, D.J., Hubbard, R.E., Jiang, J.S., Lange, G., Roberts, S.M., Todd, R.J., Adair, J.R., Emtage, J.S., King, D.J., and *et al.* (1992). Crystal structure of a chimeric Fab' fragment of an antibody binding tumour cells. *J. Mol. Biol.* **227**, 253–264.

240. Young, A.C., Valadon, P., Casadevall, A., Scharff, M.D., and Sacchettini, J.C. (1997). The three-dimensional structures of a polysaccharide binding antibody to *Cryptococcus neoformans* and its complex with a peptide from a phage display library: implications for the identification of peptide mimotopes. *J. Mol. Biol.* **274**, 622–634.

241. Pichla, S.L., Murali, R., and Burnett, R.M. (1997). The crystal structure of a Fab fragment to the melanoma-associated GD2 ganglioside. *J. Struct. Biol.* **119**, 6–16.

242. Kaminski, M.J., MacKenzie, C.R., Mooibroek, M.J., Dahms, T.E., Hirama, T., Houghton, A.N., Chapman, P.B., and Evans, S.V. (1999). The role of homophilic binding in anti-tumor antibody R24 recognition of molecular surfaces. Demonstration of an intermolecular beta-sheet interaction between vh domains. *J. Biol. Chem.* **274**, 5597–5604.

243. Otteson, E.W., Welch, W.H., and Kozel, T.R. (1994). Protein-polysaccharide interactions. A monoclonal antibody specific for the capsular polysaccharide of *Cryptococcus neoformans. J. Biol. Chem.* **269**, 1858–1864.

244. Brisson, J.R., Baumann, H., Imberty, A., Perez, S., and Jennings, H.J. (1992). Helical epitope of the group B meningococcal alpha(2–8)-linked sialic acid polysaccharide. *Biochemistry* **31**, 4996–5004.

245. Cauerhff, A., Braden, B.C., Carvalho, J.G., Aparicio, R., Polikarpov, I., Leoni, J., and Goldbaum, F.A. (2000). Three-dimensional structure of the fab from a human IgM cold agglutinin. *J. Immunol.* **165**, 6422–6428.

246. Vyas, N. (1991). Atomic features of protein-carbohydrate interactions. *Curr. Opin. Struct. Biol.* **1**, 732–740.

Chapter

FIVE

Molecular Farming Antibodies in Plants: From Antibody Engineering to Antibody Production

Rainer Fischer,[1,2] Ricarda Finnern,[1] Olga Artsaenko,[1,3] and Stefan Schillberg[1,2]

[1] *Institute for Molecular Biotechnology, Bio VII, RWTH Aachen, Worringerweg 1, 52074 Aachen, Germany*
[2] *Fraunhofer Institute for Molecular Biology and Applied Ecology, IME, Worringerweg 1, 52074 Aachen, Germany*
[3] *Current Address: Experimental Hepatology, University of Duesseldorf, 40225 Duesseldorf, Germany*

I. INTRODUCTION

Molecular farming is the production of pharmaceuticals and recombinant proteins in plants that can be cultivated on an agricultural scale. Ten years ago, antibodies were first successfully expressed in plants [1, 2] and the last decade has seen a great advance in our abilities to engineer and modify antibodies for use as diagnostic or therapeutic tools. This has been based on two critical technical developments: antibody cloning and phage display. Together, these techniques now give us the ability to generate antibodies against almost any antigen, and to reduce the side-effects of using antibodies in human therapy. For these engineered antibodies to become widely clinically useful, a production system is needed that can

Address correspondence to: Prof. Dr Rainer Fischer, Institute for Molecular Biotechnology, Bio VII, RWTH Aachen, Worringerweg 1, 52074 Aachen, Germany. Tel: +49 241 8026631; Fax: +49 241 871062; e-mail: Fischer@molbiotech.rwth-aachen.de; www.molbiotech.rwth-aachen.de;www.ime.fhg.de/

synthesize large quantities of safe, functional antibodies. Though conventional antibody expression systems, like cell cultures or microbes, are popular, they are limited. Plants offer a safer, less costly alternative that can be used to produce fully functional recombinant antibodies on an agricultural scale. Plants produce IgG antibodies that are essentially identical to those produced by hybridomas and are the premier method for the expression of multimeric antibodies, like secretory IgA. Recombinant antibodies made in plants have already been used in pre-clinical studies to treat dental caries and herpes [3, 4].

Plants offer advantages over existing systems with respect to biomass build-up, product storage and distribution and low production costs. In 1983, several laboratories demonstrated that foreign genes can be transferred into the plant genome and that fertile progeny can be regenerated that transmit the transgene through Mendelian segregation [5, 6]. Since then, many new plant varieties have been created with novel or improved agronomic features like resistance against plant pathogens, improvement of fatty acid contents or delay in fruit ripening. Plants are easy to grow and, in contrast to bacteria or animal cells, their cultivation does not require specialist equipment or toxic chemicals. Protein synthesis, secretion and chaperone-assisted protein folding plus the post-translational modification processes such as signal peptide cleavage, disulfide formation, and initial glycosylation are very similar between plant and animal cells [7–10]. These features justify the use of plants as alternative or even better source for producing recombinant antibodies at low cost while eliminating disadvantages associated with microbial or animal cell systems [1, 11]. There is interest in using plants as "bioreactors" for recombinant proteins which are currently too expensive to produce or which require significant effort to remove potential contaminants [12–15]. In many cases the production of such proteins in animal cells can accumulate to cost in the range of $10.000 to $100.000 per gram of protein. In contrast, plant genetic material is readily stored in seeds or tubers, which are extremely stable, require no special maintenance and have an almost unlimited shelf-life.

This demonstrates the promise for using plants as bioreactors for the Molecular Farming of antibodies, blood substitutes and recombinant therapeutics. We anticipate that this technology has the potential to greatly benefit human health by making safe recombinant therapeutics more widely available. Beyond the uses of plants as antibody production systems, the expressed antibodies themselves can be used to change the metabolism of the host plant, or to protect it against attack from pathogens. Importantly, modulating plant metabolic pathways could bring significant increases in the production levels of anti-cancer drugs that are currently directly extracted from plants.

In this review, we discuss the development of antibody engineering to antibody expression in plants, with attention given to the powerful combinatorial library technologies. We then focus on the current and future applications of producing antibodies in plants, how antibodies can be used to modulate plant physiology and speculate on future directions in Molecular Farming.

II. ANTIBODY ENGINEERING – OVERVIEW

The therapeutic use of antibody preparations, originally in the form of so-called "healing sera", was founded by the discovery of anti-toxic immunity by Emil

Table 1. Chronological Overview of Antibody Engineering and Plant Expression of rAb

Year	Progress	Reference
1890	First description of antibodies by Emil A. Behring	[16]
1975	Development of hybridoma technology by Köhler and Milstein	[311]
1978	First clinical study using radioimaging with anti-CEA antibodies	[312]
1982	Development of anti-idiotypic antibodies	[313]
1984	Beginning of recombinant antibody technology	[314, 315]
1985	First mouse/human chimeric antibody	[37]
1985	Development of phage-display	[168]
1987	First clinical trials of immunotoxins	[316]
1988	Expression of antibody fragments in *E. coli*	[182, 183]
1988	SCID-hu mouse	[317]
1989	Production of antibodies in transgenic plants	[1]
1990	First humanized antibody	[318]
1991	Development of phage-display technologies for rAbs	[47]
1994	Synthetic human V_L and V_H libraries (10^7)	[71, 73]
1994	Synthetic libraries with high complexities ($>10^{12}$)	[43]
1994	Development of ribosome display	[171]
1995	sIgA made in plants	[296]
1995	Expression of rAb in *Pichia pastoris*	[188]
1999	Expression of rAb using a plant viral vector	[235]

Behring [16] (Table 1). In 1975, Kohler and Milstein developed cell fusion techniques enabling the generation of cell lines that secrete a monoclonal antibody (mAb) with specificity for a single antigen [17].

Their discovery was effectively the starting point of the biotechnology industry, since mAbs could be produced by *in vitro* culture systems [17]. Antibodies derived by hybridoma technology are now widely used in medical research, diagnosis and patient management. The development of mouse mAb technology was felt by many to be the "magic bullet" sought since the time of Paul Ehrlich. However, few mouse mAbs have been licensed for human use, despite nearly twenty years of development.

The modest success of mouse monoclonal products is attributed to a number of factors. Perhaps the most important is intrinsic to mouse antibody structure. When administered to patients, mouse mAbs stimulate the production of a human anti-mouse antibody (HAMA) response. HAMA diminishes or obliterates the efficacy of the mouse antibody. A solution to the problem of developing effective immuno-therapeutics using mAbs is the preparation of human mAbs, which was problematic until recently.

Antibody engineering, using recombinant DNA and combinatorial library technologies, has created the tools for humanizing antibodies for therapeutic applications, making chimeric antibodies, isolating human antibodies and for developing antibody fragments with higher affinities and therapeutic value. Without anti-body engineering, it is conceivable that antibody expression in plants would still be unobtainable. Antibody engineering is a crucial tool for the development of plants as a production system for antibodies, using expressed antibodies to enhance the nutritional properties of plants, to engineer pathogen resistant plants and to modify plant metabolism.

Recombinant Antibodies

"Recombinant antibodies" (rAbs) is a term generally used to define polypeptides containing the antigen binding fragments of an antibody, which are expressed in a heterologous organism. Recombinant antibodies are becoming increasingly easy to produce by exploiting techniques such as phage-display libraries or bacterial expression vectors. Many forms of recombinant antibodies that have been expressed in plants are summarized in Table 2. The following sections describe the

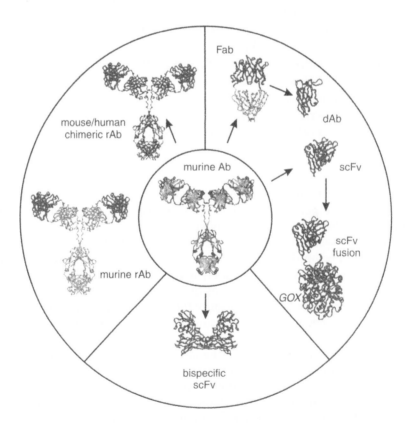

Figure 1. Forms of a recombinant antibodies (rAbs) shown as ribbon diagrams, derived from a murine IgG$_1$ monoclonal (center). (Fab) Fragment antigen binding; (scFv) single chain Fv antibody fragment; (dAb) diabody; (GOX) glucose oxidase. Images were generated using Insight II (Molecular Simulations, San Diego, CA) on a Silicon Graphics Octane workstation. (See Color plate 3)

state of the art in rAb engineering and provides many candidates for molecules that could be expressed or are being expressed by Molecular Farming in plants.

The rAb fragments most commonly used in research and therapy are single chain Fv antibody fragments (scFvs) and Fragment antigen binding (Fab) fragments. In Fab based phage-display libraries, DNA encoding the heavy chain variable (V_H) domain and the first domain of the heavy chain constant domain is inserted into a phage or phagemid vector in tandem with the light chain variable (V_L) and constant domain. In bacteria, the two polypeptide chains are produced separately and assemble spontaneously in the bacterial periplasm [18–21]. In scFv-based phage-display libraries, the V_H and V_L domains are joined by a flexible linker into a single polypeptide chain. This stabilizes the protein and ensures the equal expression of both regions in heterologous organisms. While most scFvs are monomeric, some can form higher molecular weight species, including dimers and trimers, which can complicate selection and characterization [22]. This tendency to dimerize has been exploited to create diabodies [23–25] and triabodies [25, 26]. Diabodies may be either bivalent molecules with enhanced avidity, or bispecific molecules with the ability to re-target immune effector functions, including complement fixation, antibody-dependent cell-mediated cytotoxicity and cytotoxic T-cell killing [27–33]. Diabody repertoires can also be displayed on phage and selected on antigen [34].

Recombinant antibodies are being used to target a wide variety of antigens for numerous diagnostic and therapeutic applications, such as scFvs directed against tumor-associated antigens to deliver agents such as enzymes, toxins, cytokines or isotopes for cancer treatment. Tissue-specific scFv which are able to deliver genes to cells for gene therapy applications are of high interest. All these rAb can be made by modular assembly of scFvs and other molecules and are produced and purified from bacterial and mammalian expression systems.

Antibody Humanization and Engineering through Phage Display

Recent advances in our understanding of immunoglobulin (Ig) structure combined with the recombinant cDNA approaches have resulted in the generation of recombinant antibodies (rAb) or Man-made antibodies [35, 36]. In 1985, Michael Neuberger demonstrated that it was possible to humanize mouse derived antibodies by chimerization, by replacing the murine monoclonal constant domains with the human counterpart [37, 38] and this led to the development of the technology for therapeutic purposes. Antibody engineers are now able to construct humanized or reshaped human antibodies from mouse antibodies. Starting with total RNA extracted from rodent hybridoma cells and specific DNA primer sequences, the genes encoding the Ig variable domains are cloned and sequenced. The specific sequences in the variable domains that are responsible for antigen binding, the complementarity determining regions (CDRs), are then engineered into human framework (FR) structures. These human donor FRs are specifically chosen for their sequence similarity to the mouse FRs. A three-dimensional model of the mouse antibody Fv region is used to assist in the humanization process. Critical mouse FR residues are often incorporated into the humanized antibody as a consequence of using the molecular model. A new gene corresponding to the humanized version of the rodent antibody is finally constructed, introduced into

Table 2. Recombinant Antibodies Expressed in Plants by Molecular Farming

Year	rAb format	Antigen	Cellular location	Plant organ	Transformed species	Maximum yield	Reference
1989	IgG1	Phosphonate ester	ER	Leaf	*N. tabacum*	1.3% TSP	[1]
1990	IgM	NP hapten	ER chloroplast	Leaf	*N. tabacum*		[2]
1991	V_H	Substance P (neuropeptide)	Intra- and extra-cellular	Leaf	*N. benthamiana*	1% TSP	[319]
1992	scFv	Phytochrome	Cytosol	Leaf	*N. tabacum,*	0.1% TSP	[260]
1993	IgG1 Fab	Human creatine kinase	Nucleolus	Leaf	*N. tabacum,* *A. thaliana*	1.3% TSP	[256]
1993	scFv	Phytochrome	Apoplast	Leaf	*N. tabacum*	0.5% TSP	[241]
1993	scFv	AMCV	Cytosol	Leaf	*N. benthamiana*	0.1% TSP	[240]
1994	IgG	Fungal cutinase	Apoplast	Root	*N. tabacum*	0.35% TSP	[263]
1994	IgG1	*Streptococcus mutans* adhesin	Apoplast	Leaf	*N. tabacum*	7.7 μg/ml Plant extract	[255]
1995	IgA/G	*Streptococcus mutans* adhesin	Apoplast	Leaf	*N. tabacum*	500 μg/g FW	[296]
1995	IgG	TMV	Apoplast	Leaf	*N. tabacum*	0.3% TSP	[254]
1996	scFv	Cutinase	ER	Leaf	*N. tabacum*	1% TSP	[261]
1996	IgM	RKN secretion	Apoplast	Leaf Root	*N. tabacum*	0.01% TSP 0.003% TSP	[252]
1996	scFv	BNYVV	Apoplast	Leaf	*N. benthamiana*	0.1% TSP	[320]
1996	scFv	Human creatine kinase	Cytoplasm ER	Leaf	*N. tabacum*	0.01% TSP	[321]
1996	IgG1 Fab	Human creatine kinase	Apoplast	Leaf	*A. thaliana*	11%–13% ICF protein	[253]
1997	scFv	β-1,4-endoglucanase	Cytosol	Root	*S. tuberosum*	0.3% TSP	[262]

Year	Format	Target	Localization	Plant	Tissue	Yield	Ref
1997	scFv	Oxazolone	ER	N. tabacum	Leaf	4% TSP	[259]
1997	scFv	Oxazolone	ER	N. tabacum	Seed	2.6% TSP	
1997	scFv	Abscisic acid	ER	N. tabacum	Leaf	6.8% TSP	[265]
1997	scFv	Abscisic acid	ER	N. tabacum	Seed	4% TSP	[244]
1998	scFv	Oxazolone	ER	S. tuberosum	Tuber	2% TSP	[4]
1998	Humanized IgG1	HSV-2	Secretory pathway	Glycine max	Plant		
1998	mAb	Colon cancer antigen	Apoplast	N. benthamiana	Leaf	940 µg/g FW	[248]
1998	scFv	TMV	Apoplast	N. tabacum	Leaf	0.006% TSP	[239]
1998	scFv	Atrazine	Apoplast	N. tabacum	Leaf	0.014% TSP	[280]
1998	scFv	Dihydro-flavonol 4-reductase	Cytosol	P. hybrida	Leaf	1% TSP	[243]
1999	scFv	38C13 mouse B cell lymphoma	Apoplast	N. benthamiana	Leaf		[235]
1999	biscFv	TMV	ER apoplast	N. tabacum	Leaf	1.65% TSP 0.064% TSP	[238]
2000	scFv	TMV	Apoplast, membrane	N. tabacum	Leaf	8.9 µg/g FW	[237]

(ER) endoplasmic reticulum; (TSP) total soluble protein; (ICF) Intra-cellular fluid; (AMCV) Artichoke mottle crinkle virus; (TMV) tobacco mosaic virus; (RKN) root knot nematode; (BNYVV) beet nectrotic yellow vein virus; (HSV-2) herpes simplex virus-2; (FW) fresh weight.

a suitable mammalian cell line, and the humanized antibody expressed. More than 100 antibodies have been humanized, including around 20 which have been clinically evaluated (for review see [39]).

Although humanization is often successful, it is laborious and is being superseded by the rapid, direct isolation of human antibodies from phage-display libraries or transgenic mice. High affinity human antibodies have been obtained from transgenic mice containing human antibody genes and disrupted endogenous Ig loci. Immunization leads to the production of human antibodies, which can be recovered using standard hybridoma technology [40, 41]. However, the megabase size range of the human Ig loci together with the complexity of the segmented gene structure represents an obstacle to the development of transgenic mice that utilize the full human Ig gene repertoire. Phage-display libraries offer several advantages over transgenic mice as a route to obtaining human antibodies. Human antibody phage libraries are the fastest route to obtaining human antibodies: two weeks to obtain antigen positive clones and two months to obtain a panel of well characterized antibody fragments [42].

Phage-display Vectors

Phage display of human antibody variable binding domains (V genes) has revolutionized the field of antibody engineering, since it allows the human immune system to be mirrored in bacteriophage and manipulated *in vitro* in bacteria (*Escherichia coli*). By expressing the human variable domains on the surface of filamentous bacteriophage it is possible to mimic the B lymphocyte. Similar to the B cell, the phage carries a gene for an antibody and displays this antibody molecule on its surface (Figure 2). This allows co-selection of genes encoding antibodies and the refinement of the selected antibodies toward the desired affinity, on and off rates. In some cases, phage-display libraries can be used to circumvent the need for animal immunization. Phage-display libraries can present up to 10^{12} different antibody fragments [43] on the surface of a population of phage and this diversity is critical for the successful selection of antibodies with the desired properties.

Both phage [44] and phagemid [18–21] vectors have been used for the display of antibody fragments but, generally, phage vectors have been superseded by phagemids. Phagemid vectors are small plasmids that replicate in bacteria but are incapable of forming phage particles without the addition of helper phage. Phagemids have high bacterial transformation efficiencies, are ideally suited to cloning of large repertoires, and can be formatted to direct the secretion of soluble antibody fragments without subcloning [18]. The phagemid system is based on a vector containing only the genes encoding the gene III or gene VIII proteins and bacterial and viral origins of replication. To produce phage particles, bacterial cells containing the phagemid are rescued with helper phage strains that provide all the remaining proteins needed for the generation of phage [45]. Replication of the helper phage DNA is less efficient than that of the phagemid and therefore only phagemid DNA is packed into the phage particle. However, since helper phage encodes wild-type gene III and its product (g3p), over 90% of the rescued phagemid particles display no antibody. This is a consideration when selecting large antibody libraries if all encoded antibodies in the library are to be represented. Equally important, most phagemid particles displaying antibody

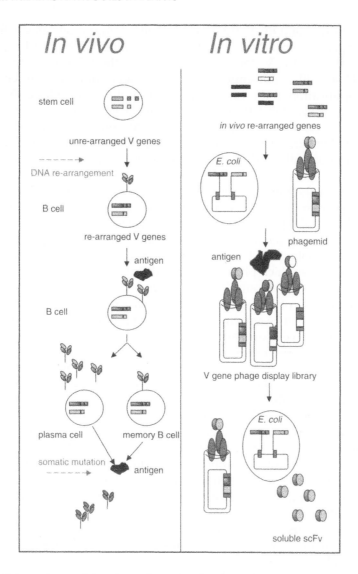

Figure 2. Comparison of *in vitro* phage-display libraries with the *in vivo* immune system. (See Color plate 4)

fragments are monovalent [20], which may be essential when selecting antibodies of higher affinity. Both scFv and Fab phage-display libraries have been shown to perform well. Purification and detection of scFv is normally achieved by adding short tag sequences (e.g., myc-tag, His-tag) to either the N-terminus or the C-terminus [18, 46].

Phage-display Libraries

A major goal of antibody engineers is to develop phage antibody display libraries of large size and diversity to permit isolation of antibodies with desired specificities, among them antibodies with high affinity. An important determinant of the composition and diversity of these *in vitro* immune systems is the source of antibody genes used as building blocks to construct the library. Libraries may be assembled from the V domains expressed by the B-lymphocytes, either of immune [42, 47, 48] or non-immune [49–51] background. This can be achieved by PCR-amplification of the variable genes from B-lymphocytes cDNA (primer sets for mouse see [52–54] or humans see MRC-Vbase: http://www.mrc-cpe.cam.ac.uk/imt-doc/public/INTRO.html). Alternatively, antibody genes can be constructed *in vitro* by gene synthesis using "randomized wobble" primers or a combination of both methods. To screen these antibody libraries containing millions of different clones, a selection system is required that has a similar efficiency to that of the immune system. By analogy to the expression of the IgM antigen receptor on the surface of inactivate B-lymphocytes, this can be achieved by displaying antibody fragments on the surface of bacteriophage or micro-organisms containing the antibody gene. Examples of these organisms are filamentous bacteriophage (M13) [55], bacteria [56] or yeast. Surface display generates a particle which physically links the antigen binding activity and the antibody genes. Using the affinity to the antigen, a specific binder can be identified out of millions of non-specific antibody fragments. Specific clones binding to an antigen can then be amplified and used to produce the antibody fragment in microbes, animal cells or plants.

Phage-display libraries can be derived from donors immunized with the target antigen, from naïve non-immune, semi-synthetic and synthetic sources. Non-immune libraries have the following advantages: (i) no immunized donor is required; (ii) a single library, if sufficiently large and diverse, can be used for the selection on almost any antigen; (iii) antibodies can be selected against self, non-immunogenic and toxic antigens and (iv) antibody generation takes less than two weeks. The major disadvantages are that (i) very large ($> 10^8$) libraries have to be generated in order to isolate antibodies with higher affinities and (ii) the exact nature of the cloned V gene repertoire is largely unknown and uncontrollable. So far, all naïve non-immune libraries have been cloned in phagemids and made from human donors [49–51].

The tissue source used to construct the library influences the composition of the library. The pool of re-arranged and expressed V gene segments from peripheral blood cells (PBCs) or bone marrow differs from that of secondary lymphoid organs such as tonsil and lymph nodes. Obviously, *in vivo* antibody repertoire selection and choice of tissue for cloning of V genes are mirrored in the diversity of the a naïve antibody phage-display library. Phage displayed antibody libraries made from donors can generate antibodies with high affinity and specificity. In addition, these libraries may be useful in understanding the humoral immune response in disease states [42, 54, 55, 57–61].

Immune libraries have two major advantages: (i) they are highly biased towards V genes that encode antibodies against the immunogen (especially if IgG specific primers are used), which means that specific binders can be successfully selected from relatively small (10^5) libraries and (ii) many of the genes will encode affinity-matured antibodies. However, there are several drawbacks: (i) there is little, if any, control over the immune response, which can lead to no antibodies with the desired characteristics; (ii) tolerance mechanisms can make it difficult to isolate antibodies against self antigens (many of which are attractive therapeutic agents);

(iii) toxic molecules can kill the potential donor and (iv) over-panning can lead to loss of high-affinity binders. In addition, if human antibodies are required, even if an immune human donor is available there are typically only small numbers of B-cells or plasma cells making antibodies against the immunogen circulating in the peripheral blood and neither bone marrow nor other lymphoid tissues can be obtained with ease. A practical shortcoming of immune libraries is that a new phage antibody library has to be constructed for every antigen and this can take up to six months. However, this is frequently faster than B-cell immortalization. In contrast to generating human antibodies, animal donors can be actively immunized with the antigen. Mice are the most frequently used donors [47], but rabbits [62, 63], camels [64, 65], cows [66] and chickens [67, 68] have been used.

Library performance is demonstrably improved by increased size and diversity. However, other factors, including expression levels, folding, and toxicity to *E. coli*, may all reduce the functional repertoire size. Moreover, some scaffolds may be better suited to form antigen binders than others, as exemplified by the large differences in V gene usage both *in vivo* and in phage repertoires [43].

Another approach to create diverse libraries employs cloned germline V gene segments [69] to which randomized CDR3 and J regions are fused *in vitro* by PCR to create semi-synthetic libraries [70–72]. The rationale behind this approach is that the diversity of these "semi-synthetic" libraries is less constrained by the forces of selection acting in the natural immune system. In the first such library, fully randomized CDR3 regions (4–15 residues) and a J_H region were appended to 49 human germline V_H gene segments. These semi-synthetic V_H regions were combined with a single V_L gene and expressed as g3p fusions on the phage surface [71, 72]. These libraries have yielded many antibodies against different antigens, including cell surface markers, auto-antigens and foreign targets [70, 71, 73], but their affinities are typically in the micromolar range.

To further increase library size and diversity for isolating higher affinity antibodies the diversity of the light chain repertoire was increased [43]. Twenty six human germline Vκ and 21 germline Vλ segments were assembled into complete V genes by PCR with CDR loops partially randomized to mimic the diversity generated by V/J gene re-arrangement *in vivo*. The heavy and light chain V gene repertoires were combined on a phage vector in bacteria using the Cre-*lox* site-specific recombination system to create a repertoire of Fab fragments of 6.5×10^{12}. High-affinity antibodies (up to 1 nM) against several antigens were isolated from this library [43, 74–76].

It is both possible and desirable to select multiple different antibodies to the same target that bind via different epitopes. Although the primary screen is often enzyme-linked immunosorbent assay, ELISA, other criteria should be incorporated into the screen, for example, neutralization, immuno-cytochemistry, or western blotting. Finally, selected antibodies should be converted to the final working format and re-assayed as soon as feasible.

Second Generation Phage-display Libraries

Selection from large primary libraries ordinarily results in a number of different antibodies with affinities between sub-nanomolar and sub-micromolar [43, 50, 74–76]. These antibodies will be well suited for most purposes, but for clinical use and commercial considerations it may be necessary to improve these first generation antibodies. This can be achieved by construction, selection and screening of secondary phage-display libraries that are constructed on the backbone of a lead or candidate antibody. Higher affinity binders have been selected from libraries of mutants diversified at the heavy and/or light chain CDR3 [77–79] or extended to other CDRs [78, 80]. A detailed study of the sequence diversity of human antibodies created in the primary and secondary immune responses also suggests other key residues for potential affinity maturation [81, 82]. Using randomized codons, a complete library with only six randomized codons would have to contain 2.5×10^9 clones [83]. Several strategies have been developed to reduce this burden including codon-based mutagenesis [84, 85] and parsimonious mutagenesis [86]. Affinity maturation can also be performed by using a bacterial mutator strain (*E. coli mut*D5) [87] between selections or DNA shuffling [88].

Selection and Screening Procedures

Phage-display libraries contain a great diversity and a great number of rAbs, so the selection procedure used is critical to exploiting this technology [89]. The antigen is used to isolate rAbs from more than 10^9 expressing clones by bio-panning. Standard solid phase panning uses antigens coated either directly or indirectly (e.g., using streptavidin) onto plastic surfaces (plates or immunotubes), and in solution phase panning, antigens are biotinylated and coupled to streptavidin-coated paramagnetic beads as a solid support. Selections can also be carried out with whole cells, tissues or even living organisms.

During selection, the antigen is incubated with the phage-display library and specifically bound phage are eluted after washing. On average, the enrichment factor is two to three orders of magnitude. Thus, several rounds of selection are normally carried out, amplifying the eluted phage in *E. coli* after each round. Positive clones are detected directly by phage ELISA using antibodies specific for viral coat proteins. In case of antibody fragments, special phagemid vectors are used, which contain an amber mutation between antibody fragment and gene III [18]. By expression of the proteins in non-suppressor *E. coli* strains, the protein of interest is synthesized without the gene III product in a soluble form and secreted into the culture medium or periplasmic space. Supernatants of single colonies can therefore be directly screened for the presence of antigen binding antibody fragments.

For many routine applications, selections can be performed very simply and effectively by panning phage on antigen coated immunotubes [51]. However, there are several disadvantages: (i) purified antigen is required; (ii) antibodies isolated sometimes fail to bind native protein antigen; (iii) it is difficult to select for high-affinity clones due to the avidity effects and (iv) it is difficult to discriminate between clones of similar affinity.

Some of these problems can be addressed by selection using biotinylated antigen in solution which allows capture on streptavidin-coated paramagnetic beads [90] due to the high binding affinity of biotin for streptavidin. The antigen concentration should be reduced close to or below the expected K_D of the selected antibody. It is also important to elute the highest affinity phage, which may require increasingly stringent eluants as affinity increases [79]. Alternatively, phage can be released by trypsin digestion, reducing agent or direct addition of *E. coli*.

For the selection of high-affinity binders from phage-display libraries, it is important that the highest affinity antibodies are eluted from the antigen. Surface plasmon resonance can be used to identify the most efficient eluant. Schier *et al.* showed that an scFv recognizing the c-erb B2 antigen could be identified with a K_D of 1×10^{-9} [79].

Selection of antibodies against cell surface markers

Identifying antibodies that recognize tumor surface markers is an attractive approach for developing therapeutic anti-cancer antibodies. Selection of antibodies against cell surface markers is more problematic than panning libraries using pure antigen, since phage displaying rAbs specific to non-target antigens are frequently preferentially enriched. Furthermore, many antigens of interest are present at very low densities, making selection difficult. Depletion and/or subtraction methods can be used to solve the first problem [91, 92], while in some cases "pathfinder" selection [93] may bypass both these problems. Pathfinder selection uses a ligand or antibody-peroxidase conjugate to direct the deposition of biotin-tyramine free radicals within a very local area. If phage antibodies are binding to this area they will be biotinylated and can be enriched on streptavidin magnetic beads. This might be very useful for the selection against cell surface marker.

Selection using flow cytometry

The combination of flow cytometry and phage antibody display libraries represents a particularly powerful method to directly select rAbs against cell surface structures in their native configuration [73]. In this strategy, heterogenous populations of cells are incubated with the phage library, allowing individual antibody expressing phages to bind to the cells. Non-bound phages are removed by washing and the cell population of interest is stained with one or more fluorophore-labeled antibodies. The fluorophore-labeled cells and attached phages are isolated using a fluorescence activated cell sorter, and the bound phages eluted from the sorted cells are expanded as individual libraries and used in additional rounds of selection before testing individual clones for their specificity. The non-selected cells in the mixture appear to remove phages that bind to structures shared by the target and absorber cells, in effect providing a subtraction at the protein level. This approach might be useful for the isolation of antibodies against very rare populations of cells such as hematopoietic stem cells in bone marrow and antibodies against non-immunogenic structures, including putative tumor-specific antigens present on malignanT-cells [94].

Therapeutic rAbs

Antibodies can be engineered so that they are more effective in therapy, by genetically fusing effector functions, radioligands or toxins to the rAbs to create tumor-specific immunotoxins. Immuno-targeting utilizes the affinity of the antibody part of the fusion protein to increase the concentration/activity of the heterologous fusion part at sites where antigen is present. An advantage of rAb fragments is their small size, facilitating tissue penetration, biodistribution and blood clearance. However, it has been shown that somewhat larger molecules (50–80 kDa) show in some cases even better pharmacokinetics and that di- or multivalent molecules increase the functional affinity and thereby tissue targeting [95–97]. Bispecific antibodies have two antigen specificities and can be used to independently bind a tumor cell and then recruit cytotoxic or T-helper cells mediating the cellular immune response.

Immunotoxins, immunoconjugates and radio-labeled antibodies

Immunotoxins are chimeric molecules comprising a cell binding activity, such as an antibody or ligand, linked to a toxin or its subunit (for review see [98]). Over the past two decades clinical evaluation of immunotoxins has been hampered by problems of immunogenicity, which often precludes multiple dosing, and by toxicity, which is sometimes life-threatening. Human enzymes, such as nucleases, are being explored as potentially less immunogenic toxins. Small toxic molecules have been conjugated to antibodies as an alternative to protein toxins. These include calicheamicins [99] and maytansinoids [100], which are 100–1000-fold more toxic than conventional chemotherapeutic drugs.

Radio-labeled antibodies are useful for tumor imaging *in vivo*. Antibodies are commonly radio-labeled by coupling radionuclides (^{99m}Tc, ^{125}I, ^{135}I) to solvent accessible lysine or tyrosine residues. This leads to heterogeneous populations of molecules and risks impairing antigen binding, as tyrosines are very common in CDRs. An elegant way to define the site of attachment of the radionuclide is accomplished by fusing a Gly$_4$Cys chelation site for ^{99m}Tc to the carboxyl terminus of the protein of interest [101].

Immunoliposomes

Liposomes are artificial lipid vesicles and the therapeutic potential of liposomes for the delivery of drugs, toxins and DNA has long been appreciated. However, the use of liposomes in clinical practice has been hampered by their poor stability and rapid clearance from circulation. Technological innovations have revitalized interest in liposomes as therapeutic agents [102]. Liposomes can be targeted to specific tissues by the attachment of antibody or ligand. The construction of sterically stabilized immunoliposomes [103, 104] has been greatly facilitated by high level expression of humanized Fab fragments in *E. coli* [105]. Fab fragments are easily attached through their free thiol group to liposomes containing a maleimide-derivatized lipid [103] or polyethylene glycol [104].

Recombinant antibody multivalency

Multivalency is a general mechanism that nature exploits to increase the interaction energy between biomolecules. A multivalent protein which can make contact with more than one site will bind with a greater free energy than one with a single valency. Moreover, at low concentrations, such a multivalent protein will accumulate – at equilibrium – at those locations where the density of binding sites is highest.

The normal function of antibodies in the immune response is to bind to the surface of a bacterium, a virus or other pathogens and then to trigger biological effects through the antibody Fc domain. This principle of multivalency is used by the natural antibodies of all classes. This is most evident in pentameric IgM, the first molecule secreted in the immune response that carries ten binding sites [106] in a relatively stiff assembly, as IgM molecules do not have a flexible hinge peptide [107]. At this stage, somatic mutation has not yet taken place [108] and the individual binding interaction is weak (micromolar). In the later course of the immune response, improvement in intrinsic affinity through somatic mutations is accompanied by class switching [109] and for most classes, the number of binding sites is reduced to two, probably because other design considerations of the molecule such as Ig class-specific responses, segmental flexibility, tissue penetration, serum lifetime take priority over the number of antigen binding sites. Nevertheless, bivalency is maintained at all times. A collection of bivalent antibodies recognizing two epitopes can also aggregate the antigen and this may be of importance in the defense against viral diseases.

Dimeric antibody fragments

For medical applications such as targeting to tumor-associated antigens, efficient tissue penetration must be combined with avidity, and fragments must be sufficiently stable against denaturation or proteolysis until they have reached the tumor site in the human body. An Ig based structure should combine small size and high functional affinity [110]. To confer the ability to heterologously expressed antibody fragments to bind at least bivalently, a variety of formats and protein designs have been investigated, such as diabodies [23], mini-antibodies [111–114] and disulfide-linked fragments [115–122].

Mini-antibodies

The term mini-antibody describes fusion proteins containing a scFv fragment fused to an association domain consisting of a long and flexible hinge sequence followed by a self-associating secondary structure and an optional cystein containing tail. The use of a hinge region creates a spacing, hinge bending and rotational freedom of the associated scFv fragments similar to the Fab arms of a complete antibody [123, 124], but with a fraction of its molecular weight. This was achieved by not adding the dimerization handle directly to the scFv fragment, but rather separating it by the upper hinge from murine or human IgG3. Hu et al. [125] showed that the mini-antibody can be expressed in Sp2/0 cells and a readily prepared version forms a disulfide-linked dimer by virtue of the C_H3 domain and a cysteine-rich linker. Mini-antibodies have proved to be excellent imaging agents in tumor-bearing mice [125].

The rAb multimerization

A variety of self-associating secondary structures such as helix bundles [111, 112] or coiled-coils (leucine zippers) [111, 112, 126–129] have also been fused to scFv antibody fragments. Certain scFv fragments, depending both on the V_H/V_L

interface and the linker length, can spontaneously dimerize or even multimerize [22, 92, 130–132]. The percentage of monomer is directly proportional to the length of the linker, connecting the two variable domains. An alternative route to dimeric and thus bivalent fragments with enhanced functional affinity is the *in vitro* formation of an inter-domain disulfide bridge by the oxidation of additional C-terminal cysteines. This strategy was shown to work for scFv-cys [133–135] or for Fab fragments [105, 136].

The oligomerization state of a mini-antibody is only governed by the properties of the self-association domain and is not restricted to dimers. Small tetramerizing polypeptides have been described [137, 138] and can be used as association domains, exploiting the potential of even higher valencies.

Nature provides us with numerous examples of molecules with low-affinity binding sites, yet capable of high-avidity interactions with their targets due to multivalent binding. For instance, the low affinity of IgM produced during the primary immune response is compensated by its pentameric structure resulting in a high avidity toward repetitive antigenic determinants present on the surface of bacteria and viruses. Terskikh *et al.* [139] described the construction of a pentameric molecule by fusing a short peptide ligand via a semi-rigid hinge region with the coiled-coil assembly domain of the cartilage oligomeric matrix protein.

Bispecific Antibodies

The challenge of bringing two different antigen-binding sites together is directly related to the problem of designing multivalent rAbs and of coupling the humoral and cellular immune response [140]. The most popular application of the bispecific antibody concept has been in tumor therapy, where a bi-specific molecule contains a tumor-binding domain and a domain to recruit effector cells to kill the tumor [33, 141–149]. As an example, bispecific molecules can bind a tumor cell and cytotoxic or T-helper cells and trigger the desired biological response exclusively close to the tumor site. Bispecific antibodies containing an Fc region are likely to be preferred over antibody fragments, for some clinical applications, in order to obtain long serum half-life and/or to recruit effector functions. For example antibody heavy chains have been engineered for heterodimerization using sterically complementary mutations at the C_H3 domain interface [150]. A "knob" mutation was first created by the replacement of a small residue by a large one (Thr366 −> Trp). The hole was created by replacing a larger residue in the C_H3 domain with a smaller one (Tyr407 −> Thr). "Knobs into holes" engineering permitted the production of an antibody immuno-adhesin hybrid with > 90% mutant yield [150].

The preferred format of a bispecific molecule obviously depends on the type of application and the amount needed. Since Fc parts are usually undesired because of concerns about Fc-dependent targeting, no glycosylation needs to be present in the molecule, and microbial expression would be the preferred production method. For *in vivo* applications in tumor therapy, the rAbs should have a long half-life in the circulation to reach the tumor site, which can take 10 h in humans [151]. Concurrently, the serum clearance rate determines the maximal serum concentration [152], the tumor penetration rate, the build-up on the tumor [28, 135, 153–155], the functional affinity and the residence time on the antigen-carrying cells.

There is a choice about the fragments to be linked (Fab vs. scFv) and there are a number of different linking technologies available. While Fab fragments may appear to be more stable against thermal denaturation at 37 °C [156] than scFv-based constructs, there is much effort in elucidating the structural basis of anti-body stability and improving the stability of scFv fragments by molecular evolution [65, 157, 158]. Clearly, scFv-based designs are more versatile, smaller and offer the possibility of combining bivalency and bispecificity.

Intrabodies

The intracellular expression of antibody fragments in eukaryotic cells (intra-bodies) is an interesting approach for research and therapy [159]. By adding various signal sequences to the rAb, intrabodies can be directed to different cellular com-partments (cytoplasm, nucleus, mitochondria, ER).

Specific binding of an engineered antibody to its cellular antigen may lead to a partial or complete inactivation of the target depending on the antibody accumulation levels and its intracellular location. This strategy was used to neutralize p21ras proto-oncogene protein in mammalian cells. It was shown that anti-p21ras scFv antibodies aggregated in the cytoplasm of the trans-formed cells and sequestered the p21ras antigen in these aggregates. This co-segregation led to the diverting of the antigen from its normal location and to an efficient inhibition of DNA synthesis [160, 161]. In addition, inactivation of the ras-protein specifically promoted apoptosis *in vitro* in human cancer cells [162]. Intracellularly expressed scFvs were also successfully used to inhibit HIV replication in transfected human cells. An scFv antibody derived from a human monoclonal antibody that recognizes the CD4 binding region of the human HIV-1 envelope protein, has been stably expressed as an ER-retained protein and is not toxic to the cells. The antibody was shown to bind to the envelope protein within the cell and to inhibit processing of the envelope precursor and syncytia formation. The infectivity of the HIV-1 particles produced by cells that express the scFv was substantially reduced [163]. Zhou *et al.* [164] demonstrated inhibition of HIV replication up to 99% in cells transfected with anti-HIV-1 gp41 scFv targeted to the ER or trans-Golgi network. They also reported that the expression of an scFv to p17 in the cytoplasm or nucleus inhibited HIV replication; in addition, the degree of inhibition was related to the intracellular targeting site [165]. The results of these studies have important implications for the development of a clinically relevant gene therapy for the treatment of HIV-1 infection.

Binding and association of rAb with its antigen can stabilize and even restore functions of the target host molecule. de Fromentel *et al.* [166] reported restoration of the transcriptional activity of p53 mutants essential for tumor suppression upon anti-p53 scFv binding in human tumor cells. This novel class of transcrip-tion-activating-antibodies is referred by the others as "trabodies". The trabodies technology could be useful to any cell type in which a disease-related protein could be the target of specific antibodies [167]. The development of a new class of catalytic antibodies and bifunctional fusion proteins provides a possibility to engineer novel functions and phenotypes.

Ribosome Display

As discussed earlier, a major focus in molecular biology and biotechnology today is the construction of large protein and peptide libraries that are screened to identify ligands with affinity to a target molecule. The key to exploiting these libraries is the physical linkage between individual proteins or peptides (phenotype) and the genetic information encoding them (genotype). Several methods based on living systems are described and in use today, such as the display of molecules on the surface of phages [55, 168], bacteria [169], yeast and animal viruses [170].

Ribosome display is a new technique for protein and antibody engineering that makes it possible to generate very large protein or peptide libraries on the surface of ribosomes, screen the library for binding affinities to a specific target molecule (ligand) and directly obtain the genetic information encoding the protein with the most desired biological function. As a complete *in vitro* system, ribosome display is the first selection system which requires no living cells. This gives ribosome display several potential advantages over phage display, which is today the preferred method for the construction and screening of protein libraries.

The ribosome display technology for linking the phenotype and genotype in a selectable particle was modeled on a polysome display system for the selection of peptides [171]. It is based on the finding that in cell-free systems in the absence of a stop codon, nascent proteins remain associated with their corresponding mRNA as a stable ternary polypeptide–ribosome–mRNA complex [172, 173]. These complexes can be used for the selection of antibodies using an antigen, if the complexes are assembled using an mRNA library that encodes antibody fragments. The simultaneously captured mRNA can then be used as template for a single step RT–PCR to generate and amplify cDNA for subsequent rounds of *in vitro* transcription/translation and affinity selection. Thus, like in phage display, antigen-binding antibodies can be enriched together with the genetic information encoding them. Due to the error rate of the *Taq*-polymerase used for the PCR-step, sequence modifications can be introduced, so that modified rAbs are generated in the next cycle of protein synthesis and selection. Since improved rAbs will compete better for antigen binding during the selection process and poorer variants will be selected against, this will result in an evolution of the selected rAb towards higher affinity for the antigen.

In phage display and other selection systems using living cells, the DNA is the information carrier for the encoded protein diversity and has to be transformed or transfected into bacteria or eukaryotic cells before each round of affinity selection, which can limit library diversity [174]. Furthermore, many promising variants may be selected against in the host environment such as toxic or inhibitory proteins or peptides. To carry out protein evolution using living systems like phage display, the PCR-amplified or PCR-modified library first has to be cloned into a replicating vector, which decreases diversity. All these diversity-limiting steps can be overcome using the ribosome-display technology so that much larger and more diverse libraries can be generated with less effort.

A typical ribosome display cycle (Figure 3) starts with the *in vitro* transcription of a DNA library to produce mRNA (step 1) for the subsequent *in vitro* translation (step 2). The *in vitro* translation, has to be performed under conditions which permit the protein to fold into the correct three-dimensional structure, while still remaining attached to the ribosome. This leads to the formation

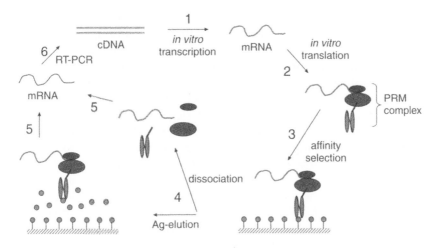

Figure 3. Ribosome display technology for the selection of rAb fragments. PRM= Protein–ribosome–mRNA complex; Ag= Antigen. (See Color plate 5)

of stable ternary complexes consisting of the polypeptide chain, the ribosome and the mRNA (step 3).

The whole translation reaction containing the PRM-complexes is then used for affinity selection (step 3) with immobilized (solid phase panning) or biotinylated ligand (solution phase panning). After stringent washing, which removes unspecific PRM complexes, either mRNA is eluted by dissociating the complexes with ethylene diamine tetraacetic acid (EDTA) (step 4 and step 5) or whole complexes are used for reverse transcription–polymerase chain reaction (RT–PCR) (step 5). During the PCR reaction (step 6), errors can be introduced due to the lack of fidelity of the *Taq*-polymerase. Where mutations and a affinity maturation is not desired, the error rate can be reduced by the use of high fidelity proofreading polymerases such as *Vent*, *Pwo* or *Pfu*. Higher error rates can be achieved by carrying out error prone PCR or gene shuffling. The PCR-amplified DNA library can now be used as template for the next round of panning.

The polysome display system introduced by Mattheakis *et al.* [171] has proven to be useful for the identification and isolation of ligands for mAb from a very large peptide library. In short, a library of DNA encoding 10^{12} random peptides was transcribed and translated *in vitro* and polysomes with nascent peptides were used for selection with mAb. The mRNA from the enriched pool of polysomes was eluted, reverse transcribed into cDNA and PCR amplified to obtain template for the next selection cycle. After four rounds of affinity selection, most clones encoded peptides specific for the antibody and showed significant homology to the known epitope [171].

A prokaryotic *in vitro*-translation systems using *E. coli* S30 extract for ribosome display of scFv fragments was described by Hanes and Plückthun [175]. They optimized the conditions for oxidative protein folding and formation of disulfide bonds during *in vitro* translation using prokaryotic extracts [176] in a model system of two scFv fragments. The effects of several compounds and conditions on the translational yield and efficiency of ribosome display were tested. The best results were obtained in the model system by adding a cocktail of chaperones, protein disulfide isomerase (PDI), vanadyl ribonucleoside complexes (VRC) and a nuclease inhibitor to the translation mixture. Different constructs were designed to test requirements for optimal transcription efficiency, transcript stability, translation efficiency and protein folding. Optimal constructs contained a 5'-stem-loop (from the upstream region of the T7 phage gene 10), a 3'-stem-loop (from a modified *E. coli* lipoprotein terminator) and a 116 amino acid spacer (derived from gene III of bacteriophage M13) fused to the C-terminus of the scFv. The stem-loops at both ends of the transcript protect against degradation by exonucleases and though stabilize the mRNA. A spacer was fused to the C-terminus of the protein to allow the protein to completely emerge from the ribosome and to give it sufficient distance not to interfere with protein folding. With the optimized system it was possible to select a specific scFv from a mixture of 1 specific scFv mRNA in 10^8 mRNAs encoding a non-specific scFv. Recently the system has been successfully used by Hanes *et al.* [177] to select and evolve high-affinity antibodies from a diverse library. Variants of a selected scFv showed a 65-fold higher affinity to the antigen than the likely scFv progenitor.

A eukaryotic system was recently described by He and Taussig [178]. They used a coupled *in vitro* transcription/translation system with rabbit reticulocyte lysate for the production of antibody-ribosome-mRNA complexes (ARM-complexes) as selection particles. The antigen-specific selection of ARM-complexes was successful without addition of chaperones, PDI or other molecules. The single-chain antibody Fv fragment used consisted of the heavy chain variable domain (V_H) linked to the complete κ light chain (K). The use of the complete light chain generates enough -distance between ribosome and nascent polypeptide chain to allow a ribosome independent folding of the antibody combining site. PCR reactions were carried out directly with the selected ARM particles without previously dissociating them. Instead, in each cycle of selection and PCR reaction a new primer was used, annealing at least 60 nt upstream of the previous one, so that the PCR product becomes progressively shorter in each cycle. However, the shortening only affects the constant domain of the light chain. The full length V_H/K can be regenerated in any cycle by recombinatorial PCR. With this constellation a 10^4–10^5-fold enrichment of the used fragment was achieved in one cycle of ribosome display which is significantly more than the reported 10^2- old enrichment with prokaryotic systems or phage display.

Ribosome display has many potential advantages over phage display and other combinatorial approaches. It remains to be seen if ribosome display will supersede phage display and the other techniques since ribosome display still needs optimization and development. In addition, new techniques for the coupling of genotype and phenotype *in vitro* have been described recently, like the direct coupling of polypeptide chain and mRNA via the antibiotic puromycin [179, 180] or the creation of man-made compartments [181]. The combination of ribosome display with gene shuffling offers a new source for the selection of novel rAbs.

III. PRODUCTION SYSTEMS–TOWARD PLANT EXPRESSION

Antibodies or fragments thereof have been expressed in a wide variety of hosts, ranging from prokaryotes such as *E. coli* [182, 183] or *Bacillus subtilis* [184], to *Saccharomyces cerevisiae* [185–187], *Pichia pastoris* [63, 188], *Trichoderma* [189], insect cells [190–193], mammalian cells [194–196] and plant cells or plants (see Tables 2 and 3 [1, 9, 10, 13, 14, 197–205]).

Expression in *E. coli*

The use of *E. coli* is convenient since cloning and genetic manipulations are carried out with this host, as are all operations with phage libraries. Compared with eukaryotes, fewer steps are needed for the manipulation of recombinant genes in *E. coli*, stable transformation of multiple copies into the host, inducible expression and characterization. Eukaryotic hosts are required, if whole antibodies are to be produced in high yields, since the Fc part carries oligosaccharide chains. For ungly-cosylated antibody constructs, however, different hosts have been considered, usually because of unsatisfactory yields in *E. coli* for the particular fragment tested.

   Antibody fragments can be produced in *E. coli* by refolding from inclusion bodies [206–210] or by functional expression by secretion to the bacterial periplasm [18, 182, 183]. Different monovalent fragments (Fv [182, 183, 211–213], Fab [214], scFv [215, 216] and disulfide-bonded Fv (dsFv)) [115] have been secreted. Several chains can be co-expressed from the same plasmid using a di-cistronic approach, which is useful not only for Fab, Fv and dsFv fragments, but also for the simultaneous expression of two chains which need to assemble in bispecific molecules. While Fab or dsFv fragments may be more stable against thermal denaturation [156], only scFv fragments [217, 218] have the advantage of being a single polypeptide, simplifying the assembly of multimeric complexes. The choice between secretion and refolding has to be guided by considerations such as expression levels, the effort to optimize a refolding procedure for a particular molecule, and the amounts or purity needed for subsequent use in scientific, diagnostic or therapeutic applications. However, the functional yield is highly dependent on the primary sequence of the antibody, and the use of engineered fragments and high cell density fermentation appears to have given the highest yields of any expression host [112, 149, 219].

Expression in *P. pastoris*

P. pastoris was originally developed as a single cell protein production system in the 1970s by Philips petroleum Co. and *Pichia* has gained widespread attention as an expression system because of its ability to express high levels of heterologous proteins (see [220, 221] for reviews). Yeast based protein expression systems are efficient and economical compared to bacterial and mammalian sources. Yeast grow rapidly, produce proteins using a eukaryote protein synthesis pathway and the cost of the media, equipment and infrastructure to culture yeast is lower than that of mammalian cells. *Pichia* can be as easily cultured and genetically manipulated as *E. coli* and has a eukaryotic secretory pathway very similar to that of mammalian cells. Eukaryotic proteins are produced in an active form and do not need refolding to provide functional molecules, as is the case for many eukaryote proteins made in *E. coli*. To date, over 120 heterologous proteins have been expressed in *Pichia* most of which are human or mammalian but the number of proteins expressed from bacterial, fungal and plant sources is growing [220, 222].

   Like other methylotrophic yeasts, *Pichia* has been widely used for the production of therapeutically relevant macromolecules [220, 221, 223, 224]. This species has gained interest compared to *S. cerevisiae* and the *Pichia* expression system is now available as a commercial kit (InVitrogen, San Diego, CA).

Table 3. Production Levels of scFvs by Expression in *Pichia pastoris*

Antigen	Yield (purification method)	Reference
Leukemia inhibitor factor	Up to 100 mg/L (IMAC)	[322]
Squamous carcinoma-epitope	10–50 mg/L (prior to purification)	[188]
Leukemia inhibitor factor	250 mg/L (DMI-Sepharose affinity)	[322]
CD7	60 mg/L (IMAC)	[323]

(IMAC) immobilised metal ion chromatography, (DMI)?

The cattle tick Mb86 antigen has been expressed in *Pichia* for manufacturing a vaccine based on this antigen and a certified production and downstream processing protocol has been described [225]. *Pichia* has been used for the successful expression of crystallization quality proteins where other approaches, such as *E. coli* based expression failed [226]. HV-2, a variant of the Hirudin blood coagulation inhibitor, has been produced to high yield (1.5 g/L) as a secreted protein in *Pichia* [226] as well as a designer cytokine consisting of a fusion of an interleukin with a soluble form of its receptor [227]. Several antibody fragments such as scFvs have been expressed at high yield in *P. pastoris* and are summarized in Table 3.

IV. MOLECULAR FARMING

The production of mAbs and rAbs is a standard technique, and the powerful tools of antibody engineering permit us to extend the usefulness of antibodies but it should be noted that the ideal expression system still has to be developed. Conventional methods are expensive or require significant effort in rAb purification. Bacteria and mammalian cell cultures are the most widely used methods while yeast or virus-infected insect cell systems play a minor role [228, 229]. These systems are limited: bacteria do not produce full-size glycosylated antibodies, contaminating endotoxins are difficult to remove from rAbs and recombinant proteins often form inclusion bodies, making labour intensive *in vitro* refolding essential. Mammalian cell cultivation can be difficult and requires expensive media additives and equipment. In downstream processing of antibodies from mammalian sources, considerable effort must be invested to remove oncogenic sequences and contaminating viruses if *in vivo* therapeutic applications are anticipated. The use of transgenic animals [230] as a source of rAbs is becoming more limited by legal and ethical restrictions.

The demands for bulk amounts of functional, active recombinant proteins, have prompted investigation of alternatives to expression in microbes and animal cells [231]. Transgenic plants [232] meet all the pre-requisites of a high level expression system [10, 233] for recombinant proteins or antibodies since plants can be grown on an agricultural scale [12–14]. Plants are easy to genetically transform and cultivate and have similar protein synthesis, secretion, folding and post-translational modification pathways to animal cells. Heterologous proteins accumulate to high levels in plant cells and plant-derived antibodies are essentially identical to those produced by hybridomas. One of the major concerns of antibody production in animal cell culture systems, co-purification of pathogens or oncogenic sequences, is entirely excluded using transgenic plants. Transgenic plants can also be used for the production of recombinant medicinal macromolecules, such as cytokines, hormones, plasma proteins and vaccines [234]. In addition, chimeric plant viruses are used for the production of vaccines [235]. Plants are easily cultivated and modern agricultural practice enables ease in scale up, rapid harvesting and processing of large quantities of leaves or seeds. To date, rAbs have been expressed in tobacco [236–241], *Arabidopsis* [242], *Petunia* [243], soybean [4] and potatoes [244].

Clearly, the impact of rAb on human health will be great but the quantities of protein required are significant. For example, according to the American Medical Association (AMA), 650,000 new cases of breast, lung and colon cancer are diagnosed in the US every year. For cancer therapy, each patient will require 10–200 mg of recombinant anti-tumor antibody, which could create a demand for up to 130 kg per year in the USA alone. It is easy to foresee that a high-level production system that is safe and economically viable is vital to this goal being realized. We anticipate that transgenic plants are the most likely system to meet this demand.

A key role for molecular farming in modern biotechnology is its ability to increase the production levels of recombinant proteins to meet the market demand and to exploit food crops as a production system. Transgenic plants offer advantages for pharmaceutical biomolecule production since plants can be grown on an almost limitless scale and the recombinant macromolecule harvested from these crops (refer to Table 4). Plants can produce high levels of safe, functional recombinant proteins and can be easily expanded to agricultural levels to meet industrial demand.

Transgenic Plant Generation

Stable plant transformation is characterized by the integration of the target gene into the host plant genome. The generation of transgenic plants uses two core technologies, *Agrobacterium* mediated gene transfer to dicots, such as pea and tobacco, or biolistic gene delivery to monocots, such as wheat and corn [245, 246]. Rice can be transformed by *Agrobacterium* and methods are being developed for other monocots. For transforming plants with *Agrobacterium* (Figure 4), the antibody gene(s) is cloned into a binary vector that can shuttle between *E. coli* and *Agrobacterium*. After plant inoculation with *Agrobacterium*, the bacteria delivers the target gene into the host cell genome itself. Transformation events are then followed by selection for cells which carry stably integrated copies of the target gene using a marker gene introduced with the antibody gene in the expression vector.

Stable transformation of plants is technically straightforward but labor intensive and time consuming. It can take 3–9 months to have plants available for functionally testing the expressed recombinant protein. This effort can be made more secure by testing the constructs and protein expression by transient expression in tobacco leaves using *Agrobacterium* infiltration [247] or viral vectors [235, 248, 249].

Antibody Production in Transgenic Plants

Antibodies are an ideal model for the expression of therapeutic or diagnostically relevant proteins in plants [197, 199, 200, 250]. Expression studies have established

Table 4. Comparison of Features of Recombinant Protein Production in Plants, Yeast and Conventional Systems

	Transgenic plants	Plant viruses	Yeast	Bacteria	Mammalian cell cultures	Transgenic animals
Risk*	unknown	unknown	unknown	yes	yes	yes
Production cost	low	low	medium	medium	high	high
Time effort	high	low	medium	low	high	high
Scale up cost	low	low	high**	high**	high**	high**
	(unlimited biomass)					
Production	worldwide	worldwide	limited	limited	limited	limited
Product yields	high	very high	high	medium	medium–high	high
Folding accuracy	high?	high?	medium	low	high	high
Product homogeneity	high?	medium	medium	low	medium	high
Multimeric protein assembly (SIgA)	yes	no	no	no	no	yes
Gene size	not limited	limited	unknown	unknown	limited	limited
Glycosylation	"correct"?	"correct"?	wrong	missing	"correct"	"correct"
Production vehicle	yes	yes	yes	yes	yes	yes
Delivery vehicle	possible	possible	no	no	no	yes
Storage	cheap/RT	cheap/−20 °C	cheap/−20 °C	cheap/−20 °C	expensive/N$_2$	?/N$_2$
Distribution	easy	easy	feasible	feasible	difficult	difficult
Ethical concerns	medium	medium	medium	medium	medium	high

* = residual viral sequences, oncogenes, endotoxins.
** = in terms of large fermenters etc.

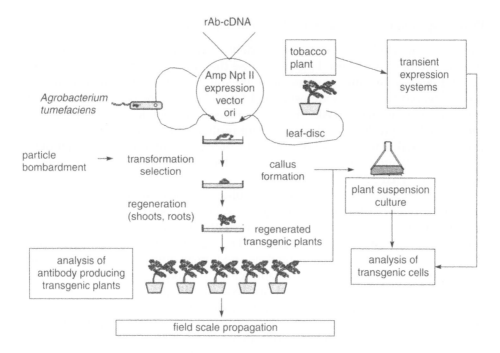

Figure 4. Transformation and generation of transgenic tobacco plants, suspension cultured cells and transiently transformed tissue for the production of recombinant proteins.

that many forms of rAb fragments can be produced. There are several technical considerations when planning transgenic plant expression of recombinant proteins [251]. Critically, the sub-cellular targeting of a rAb is an important factor in high-level expression. The pattern of codon usage in plants is different to that of animals but altering the composition of the heterologous cDNA to meet the plant pattern can improve the rate of translation and give higher yields.

The expression of functional rAbs was first reported in transgenic plants in 1989 [1] and 1990 [2]. Full-size antibodies [2, 252–255], Fab fragments [256], scFv fragments [240, 241, 257–262] and biscFv fragments [238] can be expressed in leaves and seeds of plants without loss of binding specificity or affinity. These antibodies are essentially identical to those produced by the parental monoclonal. Expression levels of different antibodies vary, with expression of full-size IgG under the control of the 35S promoter ranging from 0.35% [263] to 1.3% of the total soluble protein (TSP) in tobacco leaves [1]. This does not appear to be an upper limit, since transgenic plants have been generated with expression levels of single chain antibody fragments in leaves reaching 6.8% of the TSP [258] and up to 500 µg of sIgA per gram leaf material [264] (Table 2).

Seeds are protein rich storage organs that can be stored almost indefinitely [201, 202, 244, 258, 265] and this has been exploited to generate a rAb storage container. Single chain antibodies can reach up to 4.0% of the TSP of seed [265] and transgenic seed can be stored for up to a year at room temperature without significant losses of scFv yield or activity. Potato tubers have been used as storage containers for rAb with levels reaching 2% TSP [244].

Plant Suspension Cell Lines as a rAb Production System

Currently, plant cell cultures are not widely used to produce recombinant products of commercial interest, largely because the development of molecular farming and large-scale cultivation methods are still in their infancy and also because their potential has been underestimated [266]. Plant suspension cultures can be transferred from shake flasks into fermenters and upscaled to the 10,000 liter range [267] for production of recombinant proteins under GLP- and GMP-conditions. The goal is to increase recombinant protein yields per culture volume by increasing cell numbers (e.g., very high cell densities) while maintaining constant or even improved productivity per cell.

Based on the successful expression of a tobacco mosaic virus-specific (TMV-specific) full-size rAb belonging to the $IgG_{2b/\kappa}$ subclass in suspension cultures [268], modifications and improvements are currently under investigation including: (a) expression of other murine isotypes ($IgG_{2a/\kappa}$ and $IgG_{1/\kappa}$) as well as $IgG_{2a/\kappa}$, (b) expression of mouse-human chimeric and human antibodies, (c) expression of various rAb fragments (F(ab')$_2$, Fab, scFvs, diabodies, bispecific scFvs and scFv fusionproteins), (d) expression of rAbs with diagnostic and/or therapeutic interest, (e) increase of expression on the genetic level by modifying regulatory elements in the plant expression vector, (f) expression in different plant species with faster biomass production and reduced levels of noxious compounds, (g) pilot-scale production by using appropriate fermentation technologies (e.g., stirred tank reactor or airlift-fermenter) and (h) choice of media and addition of selective supplementation additives. Suspension cell cultures have been used for scFv production [241] and a bryodin-scFv immunotoxin [269], underlining the importance of this novel production system.

Optimization of Antibody Production in Transgenic Plants

Plants can be optimized as antibody bioreactors by exploiting the innate protein sorting and targeting mechanisms plant cells use to target endogenous proteins to organelles. Recombinant antibodies have been successfully expressed in the following plant cell sub-compartments: the intercellular space beneath the cell wall (apoplast), chloroplasts and endoplasmic reticulum (ER) [2, 202, 238, 241, 252–254, 257, 261]. Expression of rAbs in the cytoplasm has only been achieved using scFv fragments [239, 240, 260, 261]. Retaining expressed proteins within the ER currently gives the highest yield of functional protein but targeting them for secretion to the apoplast leads to significant levels of functional antibody expression. ER retention can give 10- to 100-fold increases in target protein yield compared to secretion [202]. This may be because of the presence of the molecular chaperones in the ER that promote efficient, accurate protein folding. Furthermore, rAb expression can be optimized by the use of stronger constitutive promoters in the expression vectors, tissue-specific or inducible promoters, improvement of transcript stability, translational enhancement with viral sequences and optimization of codon usage to meet the plant pattern [270].

Transgenic plants seem well suited to producing therapeutic antibodies where there will be a long-term demand for the product. A constant demand for a recombinant protein justifies investing in the large numbers of transformations required to generate sufficient (>100) independent transgenics for the selection of suitable, stable, elite lines for high level rAb production. Positional effects may explain the differences in antibody expression and transcript levels between different transformants. Selfing of the elite plant lines has shown that rAb yields can be increased 2–5-fold in certain lines presumably due to homozygosity (Fischer *et al.*, unpublished observations).

Low-level expression and additional mistargeting of antibodies to the chloroplasts of transgenic plants have also been reported by Düring *et al.* [2] using the α-amylase signal peptide. Thus, using a murine signal peptide [271] is important for efficient secretion of Igs to the intercellular space of plants, and legumin signal peptides have been used for the targeting of antibodies for secretion in plants [244, 257, 265]. The presence of a luminal binding protein in tobacco, which is homologous to the mammalian BIP, was reported [272]. This ubiquitous polypeptide binds to secretory proteins and might be essential for the correct folding of immunoglobulin V_H and V_L to form assembled functional antibodies in the plant ER. Additionally, utilization of the plant secretory pathway leads to glycosylation of the recombinant protein which might contribute to high stability in plant extracts.

Downstream Processing of rAbs from Transgenic Plants

Highly efficient purification schemes are a pre-requisite for the use of rAb for diagnostic or therapeutic uses [273–276]. Proteins must be highly purified before use, in order to minimize or even eliminate any adverse clinical reactions against contaminants during clinical uses of the proteins. In the case of diagnostics, contaminating biomolecules that could interfere with the specificity or sensitivity of the assay or degrade the reagent have to be removed to guarantee antibody activity.

Although there are established protocols available for purification of antibodies produced by animal or microbial sources, there is little available data on the purification of rAb from plants, plant suspension culture cells, leaves or seeds [277]. We established a purification protocol for full-size rAbs produced in plant cell suspension cultures [268]. Our data demonstrate that full-size antibodies can be purified from plant cell extracts on protein-A and protein-G based affinity matrices in a similar manner to antibodies purified from animal sources. A summary of purification processes suitable for full-size rAb isolation from transgenic suspension cultures or transgenic tissue is described in Figure 5, together with a scheme for analyzing the rAb. Our approach to release the antibodies secreted to the intercellular space of plant cells by partial enzymatic lysis of the cell wall was the superior method for isolation of functional antibodies. Integrating cross-flow filtration into the purification process significantly reduced time and labor for the clarification of a crude cell extract. Using affinity chromatography on a Protein-A matrix as the initial chromatographic step resulted in a very efficient removal of contaminants and a 100-fold concentration of the recombinant protein. Gel filtration served as a polishing step for the removal of rAb-dimers and for exchange of the rAbs into a suitable storage buffer. Using this approach, more than 80% of expressed full-size IgG can be recovered from suspension cultured plant cells.

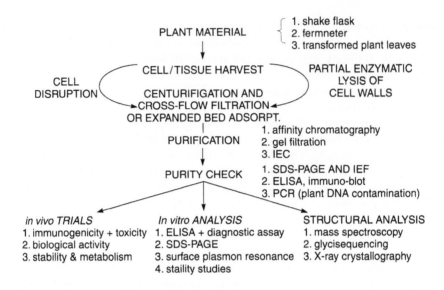

Figure 5. Downstream processing and analysis of rAb from plants. IEC: ion exchange chromatography; IEF: isoelectric focussing; SDS-PAGE: sodium dodecyl sulfate-polyacrylamide gel electrophoresis.

Characterization of rAb

Isolation and characterization of recombinant proteins from transgenic plant cells confronts unique problems because of the release of proteases and oxidizing agents (phenols, tannins) from subcellular compartments after cell disruption. Furthermore, all cell debris must be removed from the crude homogenate and a large volume has to be processed during the first downstream processing step. To circumvent these problems we have developed a protocol for full-size antibodies purification using enzymatic cell lysis, cross-flow filtration for clarification and fast-flow affinity chromatography for rapid processing (see above; [268]). Combining these techniques speeds up processing significantly and minimizes product loss during initial purification when compared to conventional isolation procedures.

Analysis of antigen-specificity and affinity of a purified plant-derived antibody demonstrated that rAb24 recognized the same neotope [254, 278] as the murine mAb24 and that the affinity constant for this epitope was also comparable. Therefore, these two antibodies should possess similar three dimensional folding, at least within the Fv-region of the expressed antibody. Investigations to ascertain a more in-depth understanding of the structural and functional properties of affinity purified TMV-specific rAbs are underway. Comparative analysis of the carbohydrate moieties between mouse and plant-derived antibodies is to be achieved by the isolation of the C_H2-domain peptide carrying the carbohydrate structure, followed by comparative mass spectroscopy and nuclear magnetic resonance-analysis (NMR-analysis). Preliminary results indicate that the N-glycosylation pattern in the plant-derived rAb24 is similar to that in mammalian cells, although there seem to be differences in the terminal sugar residues [279]. Stability *in vivo*, immunogenicity and metabolism are also being tested in mice by injecting both unlabeled and iodine-labeled mAbs and rAbs. The co-purification of plant secondary metabolites with recombinant proteins have not been extensively investigated.

V. APPLICATIONS OF ANTIBODIES EXPRESSED IN PLANTS

Plants are an ideal production system for therapeutic antibodies however, the applications of antibodies in plant biotechnology are wider than just using plant cells as a production system. Expressed antibodies can be used to modulate plant properties, increase resistance to pathogens, alter metabolic or developmental pathways and are being applied to increase the nutritional value of crops and remove environmental pollutants [12, 202, 203, 205, 280].

Metabolic Pathway Engineering

Intracellularly expressed rAb offer high potential for manipulating biological functions of the target cells [159]. The success of the application of the intracellular immunization depends on the construction of rAb that are highly specific for their targets and stable in the cellular compartment they are targeted to. Depending on the location of the corresponding antigen it may be desired to express scFvs in the cytosol or target them by means of fusion with specific targeting or retention signals into a particular cellular or membrane compartment. Expression of rAbs and antibody fragments in the cytosol of the eukaryotic cells has been reported in a number of papers. However, it has been found that cytosolic antibodies appear to be unstable. This could be due to the absence in the cytosol of chaperones that are localized in the ER and normally assist in the process of folding and assembly of an antibody molecule. In addition, the reducing environment of the cytosol does not favor the formation of disulfide bonds, thus making antibodies more sensitive to proteolytic attack [281, 282]. Different strategies can be used to improve antibody stability and solubility in the cytosol, such as engineering disulfide-free antibody domains, substituting the hydrophobic with hydrophilic residues or fusion to cytosolic proteins. Cattaneo and Biocca [283] describe possibilities to design intracellular selection schemes with appropriate selective pressures for engineering antibodies more suitable for the particular expression conditions of interest.

Antibodies targeted into the ER are usually stable and accumulate at high levels in mammalian and plant cells. If it is desirable to block a small host molecule which can permeate biological membranes, ER-targeted antibodies may be of advantage because they could provide a sink of the antigen in this compartment and prevent it from the interaction with corresponding receptors in other cellular compartments.

In view of recent advances of phage-display technology combined with improvements of plant transformation technique and increasing choice of regulatory elements for gene expression and protein-targeting, intracellular antibodies are becoming a powerful tool in basic and applied plant research. This approach is particularly suited for inhibiting functions of small regulatory molecules, because only slight reduction of their activity may lead to the dramatic changes in plant metabolism or development. Immunomodulation of the activity of a photoregulatory protein phytochrome using a cytosol-targeted scFv was shown by Owen *et al.* [260]. Phytochrome-dependent promotion of germination and photocontrol of hypocotyl elongation were both aberrant in transgenic plants, providing the "proof of principle" for the immunomodulation of plant targets.

This approach has been shown to be applicable to small non-protein regulatory molecules such as the phytohormone abscisic acid (ABA). ABA regulates a variety of developmental and physiological processes, including seed dormancy, leaf-water relations and adaptation to environmental stresses. Accumulation of an scFv antibody binding to ABA and targeted into the lumen of the ER in transgenic tobacco plants caused symptoms of ABA deficiency previously only described for ABA-deficient or -insensitive mutants. Ubiquitous expression of anti-ABA scFv led to the wilty phenotype and increased transpiration [257]. Transgenic plants expressing anti-ABA scFv under control of a strong seed-specific promoter were phenotypically similar to wild-type plants apart from their seeds. Embryo development and seed maturation of these plants differed from that of wild-type, the usual maturation programme was blocked and a vegetative programme was initiated. Anti-ABA scFv expressing embryos developed green cotyledons containing chloroplasts and accumulated photosynthetic pigments but produced less seed storage proteins and oil bodies. Anti-ABA scFv seeds germinated precociously and had reduced desiccation tolerance [265]. Interestingly, despite the high levels of total ABA (up to 10 times higher then in wild-type plants), the amount of anti-ABA scFv antibodies produced in transgenic leaves and seeds (up to 6.8% and up to 4% of TSP, respectively) was sufficient to prevent accumulation of free ABA. The mechanism proposed to explain the observed physiological effects in anti-ABA scFv transgenic plants is that capture of abscisic acid by binding to scFv antibodies in the ER may prevent its transport and interaction with ABA receptors. Moreover, the studies of the specificity of the parental mAb for ABA analogues have shown that the structure of the side chain of ABA is important for both its activity and the antibody binding. Therefore, ABA molecules bound by the anti-ABA scFv antibodies are likely to be biologically inactive.

Immunomodulation of ABA with specific antibodies demonstrates high potential of this approach for the manipulation of certain features in plants, in tissue- or temporal-specific manner. One obvious advantage over antisense technology is that one can manipulate any cellular antigen that antibodies can be obtained against, even if the complete biosynthetic pathway of the substance is not known. Modulating or mimicking enzyme activities [284] can lead to the decrease or the increase of the desired products, thus opening new perspectives for the improvement of nutritional quality, down-regulation of the toxin production and engineering disease resistance. Plant expressed antibodies recognizing small organic molecules are a potential approach for the bio-remediation of pollutants or for engineering herbicide resistance in host plants [280].

Disease Resistance

Plant diseases are a major threat to the world food supply, close to 15% of the food supply is still lost to pathogens. Antibody expression in plants offers a tool to enhance crop resistance by the expression of anti-pathogen antibodies that halt or prevent infection [236, 239, 240, 254, 285, 286]. Disease control and generation of resistant plant lines protected against a specific disease, such as a viral, bacterial and fungal infection, has been achieved in the past using conventional breeding technologies based on crossings, mutant screenings and backcrossing. Many approaches in this field have failed or the resistance obtained has been rapidly broken by the pathogen. A further limitation of conventional breeding is that it is time consuming: several generations of plants have to be screened and crossed before a stable line with the desired phenotype can be obtained and novel heterologous genes can not be introduced from other organisms. Transgenic plant technology can be used to produce transgenic plants that are intrinsically resistant to pathogens. A common approach of engineering virus resistance (pathogen-derived resistance) is the expression of viral coat protein or other viral sequences in the host plant [287, 288]. Other systems exploit transgenic plants expressing naturally occurring antiviral genes, such as ribosome-inactivating proteins [289, 290]. Resistance against fungal pathogens could be achieved by expressing enzymes that hydrolyze fungal cell walls, like chitinase or β-1,3-glucanase [291, 292].

Pathogen-specific rAb can be targeted to the cellular compartment where the pathogen is vulnerable and inactivate the pathogen by binding to its surface or to proteins necessary for its spread or replication. This strategy of intracellular immunization has successfully been used for human viruses [293], and its applications in plant biotechnology are becoming more established. The feasibility of engineering pathogen resistance by expression of rAb has been shown by different groups. Tavladoraki et al. [240] demonstrated that cytosolic expression of a scFv fragment binding to the coat protein from artichoke mottled crinkle virus caused a significant reduction of infection and delay in symptom development. Tobacco plants secreting a scFv protein against the beet necrotic yellow vein virus coat protein were partially protected against the pathogenic effects [286]. Le Gall et al. [285] have shown that transgenic tobacco shoots expressing a scFv fragment specific to the major membrane protein of the stolbur phytoplasma grew free of symptoms and flowered after two months when grafted on a stolbur phytoplasma-infected tobacco rootstock. Normal tobacco shoots showed severe stolbur symptoms during the same period and eventually died.

In our lab, the potential of using rAbs to interfere in virus infection was initially demonstrated by transforming tobacco plants with the full-size rAb24 [254]. The rAb24 has a high affinity for epitopes present only on the surface of intact TMV virions. When the TMV-specific rAb24 was secreted into the apoplast, a reduction of viral infectivity, correlating directly to the level of produced full-size antibodies was observed. Expression levels of apoplast targeted rAb24 reached 0.23% of TSP in transformed plants, resulting in a maximum reduction of 70% in viral symptoms. For two transgenic high producer lines, the offspring expressed an increased level of rAb24. Accumulation rose to 1.1% of the TSP and TMV resistance increased to 90%.

After the success of conferring viral resistance with apoplastic rAb24, we evaluated further methods to interfere in viral infection and spread. As most of these processes take place in the cytosol [294, 295], we investigated the possibility to protect plants by the expression of cytosolic antibodies. Cytosolic virus-specific scFvs are more likely to interfere with viral pathogenesis, because during mechanical inoculation only a few virions penetrate into the cytosol whereas the amount of virions in the apoplast is significantly higher ($\approx 10^6$ fold). An scFv gene was derived from the TMV-specific full-size antibody rAb24 [254]. Bioassays revealed that cytosolic expression of scFvs led to remarkably enhanced virus resistance when compared to secreted monovalent scFv24 and bivalent rAb24. Although scFv24 protein levels were very low (~1 ng/g leaf material), infectivity could be reduced by more than 90% [239]. Furthermore, upon inactivation of the N-resistance gene at elevated temperature cytosolic scFv24 expression provided systemic resistance in a significant number of transgenic tobacco plant lines (Figure 6). Recently, we have developed a novel approach for engineering disease-resistant crops by targeting anti-viral antibody fragments to the plasma membrane *in planta*. The scFv24 fusion proteins were efficiently targeted to the plasma membrane of tobacco cells by heterologous mammalian transmembrane domains and the membrane integrated scFv24 fusion proteins retained antigen binding and specificity. Transgenic plants expressing membrane targeted scFv24 fusion proteins were resistant to tobbaco mosaic virus (TMV) infection, demonstrating that membrane anchored anti-viral antibodies were functional *in vivo* offering a novel method for protecting plant cells from infection [237].

The present studies demonstrate that intracellular immunization is a powerful tool, a disadvantage might be the use of viral coat proteins as targets. Plant viral coat proteins show a broad structural diversity and this restricts the effect of the engineered antibody to a small range of viruses and under selective stress, the viral coat protein sequence can alter without loss of function. This problem can only be overcome if antibodies against evolutionary conserved domains are generated. Plants could be further protected against viral infections by expression of movement protein- or replicase/helicase-specific scFvs. Virus movement is one of the two processes that is fundamental to almost all plant viral infections, the second being viral genome replication. Antibodies directed against functional, essential, domains of these proteins should provide more potent, broad resistance against viral pathogens. Surface expression of virus-specific scFv fragments is a novel approach to shield the plant cell from an invading pathogen. Combining this strategy with cytosolic scFvs specific for conserved viral functional domains, such as movement proteins or replicases/helicases, or bispecific antibodies

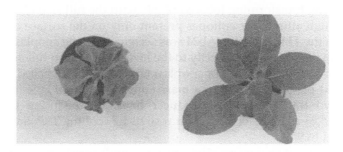

Figure 6. Phenotypes of a wild-type tobacco plant (A) and a transgenic tobacco plant expressing the cytosolic TMV-specific single chain Fv antibody scFv24 (B), after inoculation with TMV. Plants were cultivated at 30 °C and the lower leaves mechanically inoculated with 1 µg/ml TMV (8 days post inoculation) [239].

binding simultaneously to the movement proteins and replicases [238] should generate plants that have durable resistance in field.

Therapeutic Applications of Plant Derived Antibodies

Secretory IgA (sIgA) expression in plants

An interesting, relatively new idea in the field of rAb engineering is the expression of the complex sIgA in plants [296]. The sIgA is a multimeric protein that is the predominant form of Igs found in the oral cavity and at all mucosal surfaces. It is formed by two IgA Ig units containing two heavy and two light chains assembled in the conventional manner. The two Ig units are dimerized by a joining chain (J-chain) that binds covalently to the alpha V_H. Another covalently-linked protein chain, the secretory component (SC) protects the Ig from the harsh proteolytic environment in the mucosa.

In mammals, two different types of cells are involved in the production of sIgA. Plasma cells produce and secrete the 400 kD dimeric IgA (dIgA), that contains two 210 kD monomeric IgA (mIgA) Igs connected by the covalently-linked 15 kD J-chain. Epithelial cells express the SC precursor molecule on the basolateral surface. The secreted dIgA is bound by this precursor molecule, the polymeric IgA receptor (pIgR), initiating a process of endocytosis, transcytosis and proteolysis that leads to release of the 470 kD sIgA-complex into the secretion on the epithelial surface [297]. During this process the 66 kD SC as a cleavage product of the pIgR is covalently linked to the dIgA [298]. On the epithelial surfaces of the oral cavity and the gastrointestinal tract the sIgA prevents pathogens and toxins from passing through the mucosa, neutralizing them before they can enter their host or target cells.

As most infections start at the mucosal surfaces, delivering specific antibodies to these surfaces can protect against pathogens to which the host has not been exposed or become immune. In contrast to systemic diseases, mucosal diseases cannot be prevented by vaccines that stimulate systemic immunity. Vaccines stimulating active mucosal immunity have yet, beside a few exceptions, to be widely successful in humans [299]. Therefore, passive immunization using topically applied antibodies can be used to enhance resistance to infections. It has been shown that topically applied antibodies can prevent colonization of oral surfaces by pathogenic bacteria [3, 300] and penetration of the mucous layer followed by subsequent infection of target cells [299].

Topically applied antibodies can be used for the prevention of surface colonization by pathogenic bacteria. A monoclonal IgG antibody raised against the *Streptococcus mutans* cell-surface adhesin molecule SAI/II prevented bacterial adhesion and recolonization of human teeth by *S. mutans* [3]. Dental caries in humans and primates is directly related to colonization by *S. mutans* [301] and it was shown that inhibition of the colonization can lead to protection against dental caries [300].

sIgA seems most suitable of the known antibody types for topical mucosal immunotherapy. sIgA is the naturally produced form of antibody on these surfaces and is stable in this proteolytic environment [302]. The dimeric form with four antigen binding sites has increased binding avidity and a greater potential for pathogen agglutination or the formation of immune complexes. The protective role of sIgA has been shown in many systems [303]. rAb raised against pathogens of the oral cavity and the gastrointestinal tract by hybridoma technology or phage display can be engineered as sIgA and used for topical immunotherapy.

Previously used methods to produce the complex sIgA molecule were *in vitro* conjugation of SC with dimeric IgA or insertion of subcutaneous "backpack" tumors of hybridoma cells secreting monoclonal IgA [304]. Due to numerous difficulties, these methods gave insufficient amounts of sIgA and did not allow general use in topical immunotherapy. A recent publication reports the production of complete sIgA by a single mammalian cell by introduction of the gene for the processed SC [305].

In 1994, a recombinant full-size IgG with chimeric heavy chain containing gamma- and alpha-constant domains, was correctly assembled in plants and retained full binding capacity [255]. Afterwards Ma and coworkers generated transgenic plants expressing functional full-size sIgA at high concentrations [296]. To make the recombinant plants expressing sIgA, four different transgenic *N. tabacum* plant lines individually expressing either a murine κ light chain, a hybrid human-murine Ig A-G heavy chain, a murine J-chain, or a rabbit SC were generated. After sexual crossing of these plants and their filial recombinants, plants simultaneously expressing all four chains were obtained. In these transgenic plants, all four chains were assembled into high molecular weight sIgA that recognized the original epitope of the parental IgG (Guy's 13), the cell surface antigen SAI/II of *S. mutans*. In characterization studies the affinity constant of the recombinant, plant produced sIgA was similar to the parental IgG. In additional trials, it was shown that the sIgA had a three-fold longer half-life on the surface of teeth and in the saliva compared to the parental IgG. It had the same specific inhibition of *S. mutans* for re-colonization of volunteers' teeth [3].

Production of recombinant sIgA in transgenic plants opens the use of sIgA for therapeutic applications in topical immunotherapy. The sIgA from transgenic plants can be produced in large scale and used in therapeutic products. Expression in seeds or fruits of edible plants using tissue-specific promoters could provide edible protective antibodies without further need for purification. Antibody delivery through food has been shown to be successful in the oral cavities of rats [306] with IgGs and may be even more effective using the more stable sIgA. Plant produced recombinant sIgA for topical immunotherapy will be an important application for molecular farming.

Clinical trials of plant antibodies

The first clinical trial of plant-based immunotherapy was reported by Planet Biotechnology, Inc. (Mountain View, CA). The novel drug CaroRx™ is based on sIgA antibodies produced in transgenic tobacco plants and is designed to prevent the oral bacterial infection that contributes to dental carries [3]. Planet biotechnology has demonstrated that CaroRx™ can effectively eliminate *S. mutans*, the bacteria that causes tooth decay in humans and clinical trials are underway (see above [15]). Planet biotechnology is also engaged in the design and development of novel sIgA-based therapeutics to treat infectious disease and toxic conditions affecting oral, respiratory, gastrointestinal, genital and urinary mucosal surfaces and skin.

Agracetus in Middleton, Wisconsin, has created a corn line producing human antibodies at yields of 1.5 kg of pharmaceutical-quality protein per acre of corn. A pharmaceutical partner of Agracetus plans to begin injecting cancer patients with doses of up to 250 mgs of the antibody-based cancer drug purified from corn seeds. The company is also cultivating transgenic soybeans that produce humanized antibodies against herpes simplex virus 2 (HSV-2). These antibodies were shown to be efficient in preventing of vaginal HSV-2 transmission in mice. The *ex vivo* stability and *in vivo* efficacy of the plant and mammalian cell-culture produced antibodies were similar [4]. The plant-produced antibodies are likely to allow development of inexpensive method of mucosal immuno-protection against sexually transmitted disease.

The collaborative research group at Biosource (Vacaville, CA) and Stanford University has developed a technology to produce a tumor-specific vaccine for the treatment of malignancies using a plant virus transient expression system. The researchers created a modified TMV vector that encodes the idiotype-specific scFv of the immunoglobulin from the 38C13 mouse B-cell lymphoma. Infected *Nicotiana benthamiana* plants secreted high levels of secreted scFv protein to the apoplast. This antibody fragment reacted with an anti-idiotype antibody, suggesting that the plant-produced 38C13 scFv protein is properly folded. Mice vaccinated with the affinity-purified 38C13 scFv generated $>10 \mu g/ml$ anti-idiotype Igs. These mice were protected from challenge by a lethal dose of the 38C13 tumor, similar to mice immunized with the native 38C13 IgM-keyhole limpet hemocyanin conjugate vaccine [235]. This rapid production system for generating tumor-specific protein vaccines may provide a viable strategy for the treatment of non-Hodgkin's lymphoma. The goal of the therapy is to create antibodies customized for each patient that will recognize unique for this patient markers on the surface of the malignant B-cells and target the cells for destruction. Biosource plans to begin clinical trials within a year.

VI. CONSIDERATIONS FOR RECOMBINANT ANTIBODY PRODUCTION IN TRANSGENIC PLANTS

The transformation of major crop plants is now becoming more straightforward [307]. Crop plant based expression systems will become more heavily used in the near future, because they produce fewer toxic secondary metabolites than model species like tobacco, and there is an established infrastructure for crop harvesting, distribution and processing. Plants have many advantages as antibody production system, which include high level accumulation of recombinant proteins, protein folding, targeting and low production costs. These advantages are offset by the time required to generate stable transgenic lines, potential problems with gene silencing [308], minor modifications in the carbohydrates of large complex molecules [197, 251, 279] and the limited knowledge on the downstream processing of recombinant proteins from most plant sources.

Certain recombinant proteins already reach very high levels of expression, for example, apoplast targeted recombinant phytase accumulates to 14% TSP in tobacco leaves [309]. Though average expression levels of rAb in stably transformed plants are on the order of 1% TSP, advances in promoter and protein expression technology seem likely to give large improvements in production levels in the near future.

Plants are currently the premier heterologous production system for sIgA antibodies, they have significant safety advantages over classical systems for recombinant proteins in general and lower production costs (see Table 4). These features justify the use of plants as alternative, or even better source for producing recombinant proteins compared to classical microbial or animal cell systems. An important consideration is that plant genetic material can be readily stored in seeds or tubers, which are extremely stable, require no special maintenance and have a long shelf-life. In contrast to transgenic animals, both the production system and the rAb itself can be kept for long periods of time without investments in animal husbandry. It has been estimated that proteins produced in plants are 10–50-fold less expensive than those made in *E. coli* [310] and this benefit will be greater as production reaches agricultural cropping scales.

VII. CONCLUDING REMARKS

Antibody engineering and molecular farming of rAb in plants are important technologies for human health care and animal husbandry. Plants can produce hundreds of kilos of native proteins per hectare [277] and if only a fraction of this capacity can be harnessed for production of therapeutics, molecular farming has the potential to make recombinant therapeutics almost as freely available as prescription drugs for the management of human health and the diagnosis or treatment of disease. Protein and antibody engineering can generate novel, improved therapeutics and diagnostics and transgenic plants may serve as the ideal production system. As technical developments increase the level of recombinant protein that can be expressed, we speculate that the next decade will see more field trials of transgenic plants expressing molecular medicines and will be closely followed by clinical trials of the recombinant therapeutics and vaccines produced in these plants. It seems likely that we will move towards molecular farming of therapeutic antibodies becoming an economic and agricultural reality in the very near future.

ACKNOWLEDGMENTS

The authors thank Dr Kurt Hoffmann, Achim Holzem and Holger Spiegel for their contributions to the chapter.

REFERENCES

1. Hiatt, A., Cafferkey, R., and Bowdish, K. (1989). Production of antibodies in transgenic plants. *Nature* **342**, 76–78.
2. Düring, K., Hippe, S., Kreuzaler, F., and Schell, J. (1990). Synthesis and selfassembly of a functional monoclonal antibody in transgenic *Nicotiana tabacum. Plant Mol. Biol.* **15**, 281–293.
3. Ma, J.K., Hikmat, B.Y., Wycoff, K., Vine, N.D., Chargelegue, D., Yu, L., Hein, M.B., and Lehner, T. (1998). Characterization of a recombinant plant monoclonal secretory antibody and preventive immunotherapy in humans. *Nat. Med.* **4**, 601–606.
4. Zeitlin, L., Olmsted, S.S., Moench, T.R., Co, M.S., Martinell, B.J., Paradkar, V.M., Russell, D.R., Queen, C., Cone, R.A., and Whaley, K.J. (1998). A humanized monoclonal antibody produced in transgenic plants for immunoprotection of the vagina against genital herpes. *Nat. Biotechnol.* **16**, 1361–1364.

5. Fraley, R.T., Rogers, S.G., Horsch, R.B., Sanders, P.R., Flick, J.S., Adams, S.P., Bittner, M.L., Brand, L.A., Fink, C.L., Fry, J.S., Galluppi, G.R., Goldberg, S.B., Hoffmann, N.L., and Woo, S.C. (1983). Expression of bacterial genes in plant cells. *Proc. Natl. Acad. Sci. USA* **80**, 4803–4807.

6. Willmitzer, L., Depicker, A., Dhaese, P., De Greve, H., Hernalsteens, J.P., Holsters, M., Leemans, J., Otten, L., Schroder, J., Schroder, G., Zambryski, P., van Montagu, M., and Schell, J. (1983). The use of Ti-plasmids as plant-directed gene vectors. *Folia. Biol.* **29**, 106–114.

7. Faye, L., Johnson, K.D., Sturm, A., and Chrispeels, M.J. (1989). Structure, biosynthesis, and function of asparagine-linked glycans on plant glycoproteins. *Physiol. Plantarum.* **75**, 309–314.

8. Kaushal, G.P., and Elbein, A.D. (1989). Glycoprotein processing enzymes of plants, *Methods Enzymol.* **179**, 452–475.

9. Ma, J., and Hein, M. (1995). Immunotherapeutic potential of antibodies produced in plants. *Trends Biotechnol.* **13**, 522–527.

10. Ma, J., and Hein, M. (1995). Plant antibodies for Immunotherapy. *Plant Physiol.* **109**, 341–346.

11. Plückthun, A. (1991). Antibody Engineering. *Curr. Opin. Biotechnol.* **2**, 238–246.

12. Whitelam, G.C., and G., W. (1996). Antibody expression in transgenic plants. *Trends in Plant Science* **1**, 268–271.

13. Whitelam, G.C., Cockburn, B., Gandecha, A.R., and Owen, M.R.L. (1993). Heterologous protein production in transgenic plants. *Biotechnol. Genet. Eng. Rev.* **11**, 1–29.

14. Whitelam, G.C., Cockburn, W., and Owen, M.R. (1994). Antibody production in transgenic plants. *Biochem. Soc. Trans.* **22**, 940–944.

15. Larrick, J.W., Yu, L., Chen, J., Jaiswal, S., and Wycoff, K. (1998). Production of antibodies in transgenic plants. *Res. Immunol.* **149**, 603–608.

16. Behring, E., and Ktasato, S. (1890). Ueber das Zustandekommen der Diptherie-Immunitaet und der Tetanus-Immunitaet bei Thieren. *Deutsche Medizinische Wochenschrift.*

17. Köhler, G., and Milstein, C. (1975). Continuous cultures of fused cells secreting antibody of predefined specificity. *Nature* **256**, 495–497.

18. Hoogenboom, H.R., Griffiths, A.D., Johnson, K.S., Chiswell, D.J., Hudson, P., and Winter, G. (1991). Multi-subunit proteins on the surface of filamentous phage: methodologies for displaying antibody (Fab) heavy and light chains. *Nucleic Acids Res.* **19**, 4133–4137.

19. Breitling, F., Dübel, S., Seehaus, T., Klewinghaus, I., and Little, M. (1991). A surface expression vector for antibody screening. *Gene* **104**, 147–153.

20. Garrard, L.J., Yang, M., O'Connell, M.P., Kelley, R.F., and Henner, D.J. (1991). Fab assembly and enrichment in a monovalent phage display system. *Bio/Tech.* **9**, 1373–1377.

21. Barbas, C.F., Kang, A.S., Lerner, R., and Benkovic, J. (1991). Assembly of combinatorial antibody libraries on phage surfaces: The gene III site. *Proc. Natl. Acad. Sci. USA* **88**, 7978–7982.

22. Griffiths, A.D., Malmqvist, M., Marks, J.D., Bye, J.M., Embleton, M.J., McCafferty, J., Baier, M., Holliger, K.P., Gorick, B.D., Hughes-Jones, N.C., and et al. (1993). Human anti-self antibodies with high specificity from phage display libraries. *EMBO J.* **12**, 725–734.

23. Holliger, P., Prospero, T., and Winter, G. (1993). "Diabodies": Small bivalent and bispecific antibody fragments. *Proc. Natl. Acad. Sci. USA* **90**, 6444–6448.

24. Perisic, O., Webb, P.A., Holliger, P., Winter, G., and Williams, R.L. (1994). Crystal structure of a diabody, a bivalent antibody fragment. *Structure* **2**, 1217–1226.

25. Pluckthun, A., and Pack, P. (1997). New protein engineering approaches to multivalent and bispecific antibody fragments. *Immunotechnology* **3**, 83–105.

26. Iliades, P., Kortt, A.A., and Hudson, P.J. (1997). Triabodies: single chain Fv fragments without a linker form trivalent trimers. *FEBS Letters* **409**, 437–441.
27. Lawrence, L.J., Kortt, A.A., Iliades, P., Tulloch, P.A., and Hudson, P.J. (1998). Orientation of antigen binding sites in dimeric and trimeric single chain Fv antibody fragments. *FEBS Letters* **425**, 479–484.
28. Adams, G.P., Schier, R., McCall, A.M., Crawford, R.S., Wolf, E.J., Weiner, L.M., and Marks, J.D. (1998). Prolonged *in vivo* tumour retention of a human diabody targeting the extracellular domain of human HER2/neu. *Br. J. Cancer* **77**, 1405–1412.
29. Holliger, P., Brissinck, J., Williams, R.L., Thielemans, K., and Winter, G. (1996). Specific killing of lymphoma cells by cytotoxic T-cells mediated by a bispecific diabody. *Protein Engineering* **9**, 299–305.
30. Holliger, P., Wing, M., Pound, J.D., Bohlen, H. and Winter, G. (1997). Retargeting serum immunoglobulin with bispecific diabodies. *Nature Biotechn.* **15**, 632–636.
31. Holliger, P., and Riechmann, L. (1997). A conserved infection pathway for filamentous bacteriophages is suggested by the structure of the membrane penetration domain of the minor coat protein g3p from phage fd. *Structure* **5**, 265–275.
32. FitzGerald, K., Holliger, P., and Winter, G. (1997). Improved tumour targeting by disulphide stabilized diabodies expressed in *Pichia pastoris*. *Protein Eng.* **10**, 1221–1225.
33. Kontermann, R.E., Wing, M.G., and Winter, G. (1997). Complement recruitment using bispecific diabodies. *Nature Biotechn.* **15**, 629–631.
34. McGuinness, B.T., Walter, G., FitzGerald, K., Schuler, P., Mahony, W., Duncan, A.R., and Hoogenboom, H.R. (1996). Phage diabody repertoires for selection of large numbers of bispecific antibody fragments. *Nature Biotechn.* **14**, 1149–1154.
35. Larrick, J.W., and Fry, K.E. (1991). Recombinant antibodies. *Hum. Antibodies Hybridomas* **2**, 172–189.
36. Winter, G., and Milstein, C. (1991). Man-made antibodies. *Nature* **349**, 293–299.
37. Neuberger, M.S., Williams, G.T., Mitchell, E.B., Jouhal, S.S., Flanagan, J.G., and Rabbitts, T.H. (1985). A hapten-specific chimaeric IgE antibody with human physiological effector function. *Nature* **314**, 268–270.
38. Jones, P.T., Dear, P.H., Foote, J., Neuberger, M.S., and Winter, G. (1986). Replacing the complementarity-determining regions in a human antibody with those from a mouse. *Nature* **321**, 522–525.
39. Adair, J.R., and Bright, S.M. (1995). Progress with humanized antibodies – an update. *Exp. Opin. Invest. Drugs* **4**, 863–870.
40. Fishwild, D.M., O'Donnell, S.L., Bengoechea, T., Hudson, D.V., Harding, F., Bernhard, S.L., Jones, D., Kay, R.M., Higgins, K.M., Schramm, S.R., and Lonberg, N. (1996). High-avidity human IgGk monoclonal antibodies from a novel strain of minilocus transgenic mice. *Nature Biotechn* **14**, 845–851.
41. Mendez, M.J., Green, L.L., Corvalan, J.R., Jia, X.C., Maynard-Currie, C.E., Yang, X.D., Gallo, M.L., Louie, D.M., Lee, D.V., Erickson, K.L., Luna, J., Roy, C.M., Abderrahim, H., Kirschenbaum, F., Noguchi, M., Smith, D.H., Fukushima, A., Hales, J.F., Klapholz, S., Finer, M.H., Davis, C.G., Zsebo, K.M., and Jakobovits, A. (1997). Functional transplant of megabase human immunoglobulin loci recapitulates human antibody response in mice [published erratum appears in Nat Genet 1997 Aug; 16(4): 410]. *Nat. Genet.* **15**, 146–156.
42. Finnern, R., Pedrollo, E., Fisch, I., Wieslander, J., Marks, J.D., Lockwood, C.M., and Ouwehand, W.H. (1997). Human autoimmune anti-proteinase 3 scFv from a phage display library. *Clin. Exp. Immunol.* **107**, 269–281.
43. Griffiths, A.D., Williams, S.C., Hartley, O., Tomlinson, I.M., Waterhouse, P., Crosby, W.L., Kontermann, R.E., Jones, P.T., Low, N.M., Allison, T.J., Prospero, T.D., Hoogenboom, H.R., Nissim, A., Cox, J.P.L., Harrison, J.L., Zaccolo, M., Gherardi, E.,

and Winter, G. (1994). Isolation of high affinity human antibodies directly from large synthetic repertoires. *Embo. J.* **13**, 3245–3260.

44. McCafferty, J., Griffiths, A.D., Winter, G., and Chiswell, D.J. (1990). Phage antibodies: filamentous phage displaying antibody variable domains. *Nature* **348**, 552–554.

45. Vieira, J., and Messing, J. (1987). Production of single-stranded plasmid DNA. *Methods Enzymol.* **153**, 3–11.

46. Hochuli, E., Bannwarth, W., Döbeli, H., Gentz, R., and Stüber, D. (1988). Genetic approach to facilitate purification of recombinant proteins with a novel metal chelate adsorbent. *Bio/Tech.* **6**, 1321–1325.

47. Clackson, T., Hoogenboom, H.R., Griffiths, A.D., and Winter, G. (1991). Making antibody fragments using phage display libraries. *Nature* **352**, 624–628.

48. Burton, D.R., Barbas, C.F., III., Persson, M. A. A., Koenig, S., Cahnock, R.M., and Lerner, R.A. (1991). A large array of human monoclonal antibodies to type 1 human immunodeficiency virus from combinatorial libraries of asymptomatic seropositive individuals. *Proc. Natl. Acad. Sci. USA* **88**, 10134–10137.

49. Sheets, M.D., Amersdorfer, P., Finnern, R., Sargent, P., Lindqvist, E., Schier, R., Hemingsen, G., Wong, C., Gerhart, J.C., and Marks, J.D. (1998). Efficient construction of a large nonimmune phage antibody library: the production of high-affinity human single-chain antibodies to protein antigens. *Proc. Natl. Acad. Sci. USA* **95**, 6157–6162.

50. Vaughan, T.J., Williams, A.J., Prtichard, K., osbourn, J.K., Pope, A.R., Earnshaw, J.C., McCafferty, J., Hodits, R.A., Wilton, J., and Johnson, K.S. (1996). Human antibodies with sub-nanomolar affinities isolated from a large non-immunized phage display library. *Nature Biotechnol.* **14**, 309–314.

51. Marks, J.D., Griffiths, A.D., Malmqvist, M., Clackson, T.P., Bye, J.M., and Winter, G. (1992). By-passing immunization: building high affinity human antibodies by chain shuffling. *Biotechnology* (NY) **10**, 779–783.

52. Yamanaka, H.I., Kirii, Y., and Ohmoto, H. (1995). An improved phage display antibody cloning system using newly designed PCR primers optimized for Pfu DNA polymerase. *J. Biochem.* (Tokyo) **117**, 1218–1227.

53. Zhou, H., Fisher, R.J., and Papas, T.S. (1994). Optimization of primer sequences for mouse scFv repertoire display library construction. *Nucl. Acids Res.* **22**, 888–889.

54. Krebber, A., Bornhauser, S., Burmester, J., Honegger, A., Willuda, J., Bosshard, H.R., and Pluckthun, A. (1997). Reliable cloning of functional antibody variable domains from hybridomas and spleen cell repertoires employing a reengineered phage display system *J. Immunol. Methods* **201**, 35–55.

55. Winter, G., Griffiths, A.D., Hawkins, R.E., and Hoogenboom, H.R. (1994). Making antibodies by phage display technology. *Annu. Rev. Immunol.* **12**, 433–455.

56. Daugherty, P.S., Chen, G., Olsen, M.J., Iverson, B.L., and Georgiou, G. (1998). Antibody affinity maturation using bacterial surface display. *Protein Eng.* **11**, 825–832.

57. Krebber, C., Spada, S., Desplancq, D., and Pluckthun, A. (1995). Co-selection of cognate antibody-antigen pairs by selectively-infective phages. *FEBS Lett.* **377**, 227–231.

58. Griffin, H.M., and Ouwehand, W.H. (1995). A human monoclonal antibody specific for the leucine-33 (P1A1, HPA-1a) form of platelet glycoprotein IIIa from a V gene phage display library. *Blood* **86**, 4430–4436.

59. Finnern, R., Bye, J.M., Dolman, K.M., Zhao, M.-M., Short, A., Marks, J.D., Lockwood, M.C., and Ouwehand, W.H. (1995). Molecular characteristics of anti-self antibody fragments against neutrophil cytoplsmic antigens from human V gene phage display libraries. *Clin. Exp. Immunol.* **102**, 566–574.

60. Tafi, R., Bandi, R., Prezzi, C., Mondelli, M.U., Cortese, R., Monaci, P., and Nicosia, A. (1997). Identification of HCV core mimotopes: improved methods for the selection and use of disease-related phage-displayed peptides. *Biol. Chem.* **378**, 495–502.

61. Clark, M.A., Hawkins, N.J., Papaioannou, A., Fiddes, R.J., and Ward, R.L. (1997). Isolation of human anti-c-erbB-2 Fabs from a lymph node-derived phage display library. *Clin. Exp. Immunol.* **109**, 166–174.

62. Lang, I.M., Barbas, C.F., 3rd and Schleef, R.R. (1996). Recombinant rabbit Fab with binding activity to type-1 plasminogen activator inhibitor derived from a phage-display library against human alpha-granules. *Gene* **172**, 295–298.

63. Ridder, R., Schmitz, R., Legay, F., and Gram, H. (1995). Generation of rabbit monoclonal antibody fragments from a combinatorial phage display library and their production in the yeast Pichia pastoris. *Bio/Tech.* **13**, 255–260.

64. Lauwereys, M., Arbabi Ghahroudi, M., Desmyter, A., Kinne, J., Holzer, W., De Genst, E., Wyns, L., and Muyldermans, S. (1998). Potent enzyme inhibitors derived from dromedary heavy-chain antibodies. *Embo. J.* **17**, 3512–3520.

65. Davies, J., and Riechmann, L. (1996). Single antibody domains as small recognition units: design and *in vitro* antigen selection of camelized, human VH domains with improved protein stability. *Protein Eng.* **9**, 531–537.

66. O'Brien, P.M., Aitken, R., O'Neil, B.W., and Campo, M.S. (1999). Generation of native bovine mAbs by phage display. *Proc. Natl. Acad. Sci. USA* **96**, 640–645.

67. Davies, E.L., Smith, J.S., Birkett, C.R., Manser, J.M., Anderson-Dear, D.V., and Young, J.R. (1995). Selection of specific phage-display antibodies using libraries derived from chicken immunoglobulin genes. *J. Immunol.* **186**, 125–135.

68. Yamanaka, H.I., Inoue, T., and Ikeda-Tanaka, O. (1996). Chicken monoclonal antibody isolated by a phage display system. *J. Immunol.* **157**, 1156–1162.

69. Tomlinson, I.M. (1998). *Immunoglobulin genes*, Academic press, London.

70. de Kruif, J., Boel, E., and Logtenberg, T. (1995). Selection and application of human single chain Fv antibody fragments from a semi-synthetic phage antibody display library with designed CDR3 regions. *J. Mol. Biol.* **246**, 97–105.

71. Nissim, A., Hoogenboom, H.R., Tomlinson, I.M., Flynn, G., Midgley, C., Lane, D., and Winter, G. (1994). Antibody fragments from a 'single pot' phage display library as immunochemical reagents. *EMBO.* **13**, 692–698.

72. Hoogenboom, H.R., and Winter, G. (1992). By-passing immunisation. Human antibodies from synthetic repertoires of germline VH gene segments rearranged *in vitro*. *J. Mol. Biol.* **20**, 381–388.

73. de Kruif, J., Terstappen, L., Boel, E., and Logtenberg, T. (1995). Rapid selection of cell subpopulation-specific human monoclonal antibodies from a synthetic phage antibody library. *Proc. Natl. Acad. Sci. USA* **92**, 3938–3942.

74. Doorbar, J., Foo, C., Coleman, N., Medcalf, L., Hartley, O., Prospero, T., Napthine, S., Sterling, J., Winter, G., and Griffin, H. (1997). Characterization of events during the late stages of HPV16 infection *in vivo* using high-affinity synthetic Fabs to E4. *Virology* **238**, 40–52.

75. Lalla, C.d., Tamborini, E., Longhi, R., Tresoldi, E., Manoni, M., Siccardi, A.G., Arosio, P., and Sidoli, A. (1996). Human recombinant antibody fragments specific for a rye-grass pollen allergen: characterization and potential applications. *Mol. Immunol.* **33**, 1049–1058.

76. de Wildt, R.M., Finnern, R., Ouwehand, W.H., Griffiths, A.D., van Venrooij, W.J., and Hoet, R.M. (1996). Characterization of human variable domain antibody fragments against the U1 RNA-associated A protein, selected from a synthetic and patient-derived combinatorial V gene library. *Eur. J. Immunol.* **26**, 629–639.

77. Osbourn, J.K., Field, A., Wilton, J., Derbyshire, E., Earnshaw, J.C., Jones, P.T., Allen, D., and McCafferty, J. (1996). Generation of a panel of related human scFv antibodies with high affinities for human CEA. *Immunotechnology* **2**, 181–196.

78. Yang, W.P., Green, K., Pinz-Sweeney, S., Briones, A. T., Burton, D.R., and Barbas, C.F., 3rd. (1995). CDR walking mutagenesis for the affinity maturation of a potent human anti-HIV-1 antibody into the picomolar range. *J. Mol. Biol.* **254**, 392–403.

79. Schier, R., and Marks, J.D. (1996). Efficient *in vitro* affinity maturation of phage anti-bodies using BIAcore guided selections. *Hum Antibodies Hybridomas* **7**, 97–105.

80. Barbas, C.F., 3rd, Hu, D., Dunlop, N., Sawyer, L., Cababa, D., Hendry, R.M., Nara, P.L., and Burton, D.R. (1994). *In vitro* evolution of a neutralizing human antibody to human immunodeficiency virus type 1 to enhance affinity and broaden strain cross-reactivity. *Proc. Natl. Acad. Sci. USA* **91**, 3809–3813.

81. Ignatovich, O., Tomlinson, I.M., Jones, P.T., and Winter, G. (1997). The creation of diversity in the human immunoglobulin V(lambda) repertoire. *J. Mol. Biol.* **268**, 69–77.

82. Tomlinson, I.M., Walter, G., Jones, P.T., Dear, P.H., Sonnhammer, E.L., and Winter, G. (1996). The imprint of somatic hypermutation on the repertoire of human germline V genes. *J. Mol. Biol.* **256**, 813–817.

83. Clackson, T., and Wells, J.A. (1994). *In vitro* selection from protein and peptide libraries. *Trends in Biotechnology* **12**, 173–184.

84. Virnekas, B., Ge, L., Pluckthun, A., Schneider, K.C., Wellnhofer, G., and Moroney, S.E. (1994). Trinucleotide phosphoramidites: ideal reagents for the synthesis of mixed oligonucleotides for random mutagenesis. *Nucleic Acids Res.* **22**, 5600–5607.

85. Glaser, S.M., Yelton, D.E., and Huse, W.D. (1992). Antibody engineering by codon-based mutagenesis in a filamentous phage system. *J. Immunol.* **149**, 3903–3913.

86. Schier, R., Balint, R.F., McCall, A., Apell, G., Larrick, J.W., and Marks, J.D. (1996). Identification of functional and structural amino-acid residues by parsimonious mutagenesis. *Gene* **169**, 147–155.

87. Low, N.M., Holliger, P.H., and Winter, G. (1996). Mimicking somatic hypermutation: affinity maturation of antibodies displayed on bacteriophage using a bacterial mutator strain. *J. Mol. Biol.* **260**, 359–368.

88. Stemmer, W. (1994). DNA shuffling by random fragmentation and reassembly: *In vitro* recombination for molecular evolution. *Proc. Natl. Acad. Sci. USA* **91**, 10747–10751.

89. de Bruin, R., Spelt, K., Mol, J., Koes, R., and Quattrocchio, F. (1999). Selection of high-affinity phage antibodies from phage display libraries. *Nature Biotech.* **17**, 397–399.

90. Hawkins, R.E., Russell, S.J., and Winter, G. (1992). Selection of phage antibodies by binding affinity. Mimicking affinity maturation. *J. Mol. Biol.* **226**, 889–896.

91. Van Ewijk, W., de Kruif, J., Germeraad, W.T., Berendes, P., Ropke, C., Platenburg, P.P., and Logtenberg, T. (1997). Subtractive isolation of phage-displayed single-chain anti-bodies to thymic stromal cells by using intact thymic fragments. *Proc. Natl. Acad. Sci. USA* **94**, 3903–3908.

92. Marks, J.D., Ouwehand, W.H., Bye, J.M., Finnern, R., Gorick, B.D., Voak, D., Thorpe, S., Hughes-Jones, N.C., and Winter, G. (1993). Human antibody fragments specific for human blood group antigens from a phage display library. *Bio/Tech.* **11**, 1145–1149.

93. Osbourn, J.K., Derbyshire, E.J., Vaughan, T.J., Field, A.W., and Johnson, K.S. (1998). Pathfinder selection: *in situ* isolation of novel antibodies. *Immunotechnology* **3**, 293–302.

94. van der Vuurst de Vries, A., de Kruif, J., van Ewijk, W., and Logtenberg. T. (1997). *Phage antibody display libraries: a tool to search for novel cell surface markers*, Harwood academic, Amsterdam, NL.

95. Begent, R.H., and Chester, K.A. (1997). Single-chain Fv antibodies for targeting cancer therapy. *Biochem. Soc. Trans.* **25**, 715–717.

96. Begent, R.H.J., and Pedley, R.B. (1990). Antibody targeted therapy in cancer: comparison of murine and clinical studies. *Cancer Treat. Rev.* **17**, 373–378.

97. Begent, R.H.J., Verhaar, M.J., Chester, K.A., Casey, J.L., Green, A.J., Napire, M.P., Hope-Stone, L.D., Cushen, N., Keep, P.A., Johnson, C.J., Hawkins, R.E., Hilson, A.J.W., and Robson, L. (1996). Clinical evidence of efficient tumor targeting based on single-chain Fv antibody selected from a combinatorial library. *Nature Med.* **2**, 979–984.

98. Ghetie, M.-A., and Vitetta, E.S. (1994). Recent developments in immunotoxin therapy. *Curr. Opin. Immunol.* **6**, 707–714.

99. Hinman, L.M., Hamann, P.R., Wallace, R., Menendez, A.T., Durr, F.E., and Upeslacis, J. (1993). Preparation and characterization of monoclonal antibody conjugates of the calicheamicins: a novel and potent family of antitumor antibiotics. *Cancer Res.* **53**, 3336–3342.

100. Chari, R.V., Martell, B.A., Gross, J.L., Cook, S.B., Shah, S.A., Blattler, W.A., McKenzie, S.J., and Goldmacher, V.S. (1992). Immunoconjugates containing novel maytansinoids: promising anticancer drugs. *Cancer Res.* **52**, 127–131.

101. Zhong, J.J. (1995). Recent advances in cell cultures of Taxus spp. for production of the natural anticancer drug taxol. *Plant Tissue Culture and Biotechnology* **1**, 75–80.

102. Lasic, D.D., and Papahadjopoulos, D. (1995). Liposomes revisited. *Science* **267**, 1275–1276.

103. Park, J.W., Hong, K., Carter, P., Asgari, H., Guo, L.Y., Keller, G.A., Wirth, C., Shalaby, R., Kotts, C., Wood, W.I., and *et al.* (1995). Development of anti-p185HER2 immunoliposomes for cancer therapy. *Proc. Natl. Acad. Sci. USA* **92**, 1327–1331.

104. Kirpotin, D., Park, J.W., Hong, K., Zalipsky, S., Li, W.L., Carter, P., Benz, C.C., and Papahadjopoulos, D. (1997). Sterically stabilized anti-HER2 immunoliposomes: design and targeting to human breast cancer cells *in vitro. Biochemistry* **36**, 66–75.

105. Carter, P., Kelley, R.F., Rodrigues, M.L., Snedecor, B., Covarrubias, M., Velligan, M.D., Wong, W.L., Rowland, A.M., Kotts, C.E., Carver, M.E., and *et al.* (1992). High level *Escherichia coli* expression and production of a bivalent humanized antibody fragment. *Biotechnology* (N Y). **10**, 163–167.

106. Randall, T.D., Brewer, J.W., and Corley, R.B. (1992). Direct evidence that J chain regulates the polymeric structure of IgM in antibody-secreting B-cells. *J. Biol. Chem.* **267**, 18002–18007.

107. Feinstein, A., and Munn, E.A. (1969). Conformation of the free and antigen-bound IgM antibody molecules. *Nature* **224**, 1307–1309.

108. Gearhart, P.J., Johnson, N.D., Douglas, R., and Hood, L. (1981). IgG antibodies to phosphorylcholine exhibit more diversity than their IgM counterparts, *Nature* **291**, 29–34.

109. Harriman, W., Volk, H., Defranoux, N., and Wabl, M. (1993). Immunoglobulin class switch recombination. *Annu. Rev. Immunol.* **11**, 361–384.

110. Thomas, G.D., Chappell, M.J., Dykes, P.W., Ramsden, D.B., Godfrey, K.R., Ellis, J.R., and Bradwell, A.R. (1989). Effect of dose, molecular size, affinity, and protein binding on tumor uptake of antibody or ligand: a biomathematical model. *Cancer Res.* **49**, 3290–3296.

111. Pack, P., and Pluckthun, A. (1992). Miniantibodies: use of amphipathic helices to produce functional, flexibly linked dimeric FV fragments with high avidity in *Escherichia coli. Biochemistry* **31**, 1579–1584.

112. Pack, P., Kujau, M., Schroeckh, V., Knuepfer, U., Wenderoth, R., Riesenberg, D., and Plueckthun, A. (1993). Improved bivalent miniantibodies, with identical avidity as whole antibodies, produced by high cell density fermentation of *Escherichia coli. Bio/Tech.* **11**, 1271–1277.

113. Pack, P., Muller, K., Zahn, R., and Pluckthun, A. (1995). Tetravalent miniantibodies with high avidity assembling in *Escherichia coli. J. Mol. Biol.* **246**, 28–34.

114. Müller, K.M., Arndt, K.M., Strittmatter, W., and Plückthun, A. (1998). The first constant domain (C(H)1 and C(L)) of an antibody used as heterodimerization domain for bispecific miniantibodies. *FEBS Letters.* **422**, 259–264.

115. Brinkmann, U., Chowdhury, P.S., Roscoe, D.M., and Pastan, I. (1995). Phage display of disulfide-stabilized Fv fragments. *J. Immunol. Methods* **182**, 41–50.

116. Almog, O., Benhar, I., Vasmatzis, G., Tordova, M., Lee, B., Pastan, I., and Gilliland, G.L. (1998). Crystal structure of the disulfide-stabilized Fv fragment of anticancer antibody B1: conformational influence of an engineered disulfide bond. *Proteins* **31**, 128–138.

117. Benhar, I., and Pastan, I. (1995). Characterization of B1(Fv)PE38 and B1(dsFv)PE38: single-chain and disulfide-stabilized Fv immunotoxins with increased activity that cause complete remissions of established human carcinoma xenografts in nude mice. *Clin. Cancer Res.* 1, 1023–1029.
118. McCartney, J.E., Tai, M.-S., Hudziak, R.M., Adams, G.P., Weiner, L.M., Jin, D., Stafford III, W.F., Liu, S., Bookmna, M.A., Laminet, A., Fand, I., Houston, L.L., Oppermann, H., and Huston, J. S. (1995). Engineering disulfide-linked single-chain Fv dimrs (sFv')2 with improved solution and targeting properties: anti-digoxin 26–10 (sFv')2 and anti-c-erb-2741F8 (sFv')2 made by protein folding and bonded through C-terminal cysteinyl peptides. *Protein Eng.* 8, 301–314.
119. Proba, K., Ge, L., and Plückthun, A. (1995). Functional antibody single-chain fragments from the cytoplasm of *Escherichia coli*: influence of thioredoxin reductase (TrxB). *Gene* 159, 203–207.
120. Reiter, Y., Brinkmann, U., Webber, K.O., Jung, S.H., Lee, B., and Pastan, I. (1994). Engineering interchain disulfide bonds into conserved framework regions of Fv fragments: improved biochemical characteristics of recombinant immunotoxins containing disulfide-stabilized Fv. *Protein Engineering* 7, 697–704.
121. Reiter, Y., Brinkmann, U., Lee, B., and Pastan, I. (1996). Engineering antibody Fv fragments for cancer detection and therapy: disulfide-stabilized Fv fragments. *Nature Biotechnology* 14, 1239–1245.
122. Reiter, Y., Kreitman, R.J., Brinkmann, U., and Pastan, I. (1994). Cytotoxic and antitumor activity of a recombinant immunotoxin composed of disulfide-stabilized anti-Tac Fv fragment and truncated Pseudomonas exotoxin. *International Journal of Cancer* 58, 142–149.
123. Burton, D.R. (1990). Antibody: the flexible adaptor molecule. *Trends Biochem. Sci.* 15, 64–69.
124. Harris, L.J., Larson, S.B., Hasel, K.W., Day, J., Greenwood, A., and McPherson, A. (1992). The three-dimensional structure of an intact monoclonal antibody for canine lymphoma. *Nature* 360, 369–372.
125. Hu, S., Shively, L., Raubitschek, A., Sherman, M., Williams, L. E., Wong, J.Y., Shively, J.E., and Wu, A.M. (1996). Minibody: A novel engineered anti-carcinoembryonic antigen antibody fragment (single-chain Fv-CH3) which exhibits rapid, high-level targeting of xenografts. *Cancer Res.* 56, 3055–3061.
126. O'Shea, E.K., Klemm, J.D., Kim, P.S., and Alber, T. (1991). X-ray structure of the GCN4 leucine zipper, a two-stranded, parallel coiled coil. *Science* 254, 539–544.
127. O'Shea, E.K., Rutkowski, R., Stafford, W.F.d., and Kim, P.S. (1989). Preferential heterodimer formation by isolated leucine zippers from fos and jun, *Science* 245, 646–648.
128. O'Shea, E.K., Rutkowski, R., and Kim, P.S. (1989). Evidence that the leucine zipper is a coiled coil. *Science* 243, 538–542.
129. Kostelny, S.A., Cole, M.S., and Tso, J.Y. (1992). Formation of a bispecific antibody by the use of leucine zippers. *J. Immunol.* 148, 1547–1553.
130. Essig, N.Z., Wood, J.F., Howard, A.J., Raag, R., and Whitlow, M. (1993). Crystallization of single-chain Fv proteins. *J. Mol. Biol.* 234, 897–901.
131. Whitlow, M., Bell, B.A., Feng, S.-L., Filpula, D., Hardman, K.D., Hubert, S.L., Rollence, M.L., Wood, J.F., Schott, M.E., Milenic, D.E., Yokota, T., and Schlom, J. (1993). An improved linker for single-chain Fv with reduced aggregation and enhanced proteolytic stability. *Prot. Eng.* 6, 989–995.
132. Holliger, P., Prospero, T., and Winter, G. (1993). "Diabodies": small bivalent and bispecific antibody fragments. *Proc. Natl. Acad. Sci. USA* 90, 6444–6448.
133. Cumber, A.J., Ward, E.S., Winter, G., Parnell, G.D., and Wawrzynczak, E.J. (1992). Comparative stabilities *in vitro* and *in vivo* of a recombinant mouse antibody FvCys fragment and a bisFvCys conjugate. *J. Immunol.* 149, 120–126.

134. Kipriyanov, S.M., Dübel, S., Breitling, F., Kontermann, R.E., and Little, M. (1994). Recombinant single-chain Fv fragments carrying C-terminal cysteine residues: production of bivalent and biotinylated miniantibodies. *Mol. Immunol.* **31**, 1047–1058.

135. Adams, G.P., McCartney, J.E., Tai, M.-S., Oppermann, H., Huston, J.S., Stafford, W.F., Bookman, M.A., Fand, I., Houston, L.L., and Weiner, L.M. (1993). Highly specific *in vivo* tumor targeting by monovalent and divalent forms of 741F8 anti-c-erbB-2 single chain Fv. *Cancer Res.* **53**, 4026–4034.

136. Rodrigues, M.L., Snedecor, B., Chen, C., Wong, W.L.T., Garg, S., Blank, G.S., Maneval, D., and Carter, P. (1993). Engineering Fab' fragments for efficient F(ab)'2 formation in *Escherichia coli* and for improved *in vivo* stability. *J.Immunol.* **151**, 6954–6961.

137. Jeffrey, P.D., Gorina, S., and Pavletich, N.P. (1995). Crystal structure of the tetramerization domain of the p53 tumor suppressor at 1.7 angstroms. *Science* **267**, 1498–1502.

138. Harbury, P.B., Zhang, T., Kim, P.S., and Alber, T. (1993). A switch between two-, three-, and four-stranded coiled coils in GCN4 leucine zipper mutants. *Science* **262**, 1401–1407.

139. Terskikh, A.V., Le Doussal, J.M., Crameri, R., Fisch, I., Mach, J.P., and Kajava, A.V. (1997). "Peptabody": a new type of high avidity binding protein. *Proc. Natl. Acad. Sci. USA* **94**, 1663–1668.

140. George, A., and Huston, J. (1997). *Bispecific antibody engineering*, Harwood academic, Amsterdam, NL.

141. Carter, P., and Merchant, A.M. (1997). Engineering antibodies for imaging and therapy. *Curr. Opin. Biotechnol.* **8**, 449–454.

142. Gilliland, L.K., Clark, M.R., and Waldmann, H. (1988). Universal bispecific antibody for targeting tumor cells for destruction by cytotoxic T-cells. *Proc. Natl. Acad. Sci. USA* **85**, 7719–7723.

143. Barr, I.G., Miescher, S., von Fliedner, V., Buchegger, F., Barras, C., Lanzavecchia, A., Mach, J.-P., and Carrel, S. (1989). *In vivo* localization of a bispecific antibody which targets human T-lymphocytes to lyse human colon cancer cells. *Int. J. Cancer.* **43**, 501–507.

144. Cheong, H.S., Chang, J.S., Park, J.M., and M.B.S. (1990). Affinity enhancement of bispecific antibody against two different epitopes in the same antigen. *Biochem. Biophys. Res. Commun.* **173**, 795–800.

145. Snider, D.P., Kaubisch, A., and Segal, D.M. (1990). Enhanced antigen immunogenicity induced by bispecific antibodies. *J. Exp. Med.* **171**, 1957–1963.

146. Berg, J., Loetscher, E., Steimer, K.S., Capon, D.J., Baenziger, J., Jaeck, H.-M., and Wabl, M. (1991). Bispecific antibodies that mediate killing of cells infected with human immunodeficiency virus of any strain. *Proc. Natl. Acad. Sci. USA* **88**, 4723–4727.

147. Demanet, C., Brissinck, J., Moser, M., Leo, O., and Thielemans, K. (1992). Bispecific antibody therapy of two murine B-cell lymphomas. *Int. J. Cancer Suppl.* **7**, 67–68.

148. Nolan, O., and O'Kennedy, R. (1992). Bifunctional antibodies and their potential clinical applications. *Int. J. Clin. Lab. Res.* **22**, 21–27.

149. Carter, P., Ridgway, J., and Zhu, Z. (1995). Toward the production of bispecific antibody fragments for clinical applications. *Journal of Hematotherapy* **4**, 463–470.

150. Ridgway, J.B., Presta, L.G., and Carter, P. (1996). 'Knobs-into-holes' engineering of antibody CH3 domains for heavy chain heterodimerization. *Protein Eng.* **9**, 617–621.

151. Baxter, L.T., Zhu, H., Mackensen, D.G., Butler, W.F., and Jain, R.K. (1995). Biodistribution of monoclonal antibodies: scale-up from mouse to human using a physiologically based pharmacokinetic model. *Cancer Res.* **55**, 4611–4622.

152. King, D.J., Turner, A., Farnsworth, A.P., Adair, J.R., Owens, R.J., Pedley, R.B., Baldock, D., Proudfoot, K.A., Lawson, A.D., Beeley, N.R., and *et al.* (1994). Improved tumor targeting with chemically cross-linked recombinant antibody fragments. *Cancer Res.* **54**, 6176–6185.

153. Yokota, T., Milenic, D.E., Whitlow, M., and Schlom, J. (1992). Rapid tumor penetration of a single-chain Fv and comparison with other immunoglobulin forms. *Cancer Res.* **52**, 3402–3408.

154. Milenic, D.E., Yokota, T., Filpula, D.R., Finkelman, M.A., Dodd, S.W., Wood, J.F., Whitlow, M., Snoy, P., and Schlom, J. (1991). Construction, binding properties, metabolism, and tumor targeting of a single-chain Fv derived from the pancarcinoma monoclonal antibody CC49. *Cancer Res.* **51**, 6363–6371.

155. Colcher, D., Bird, R., Roselli, M., Hardman, K.D., Johnson, S., Pope, S., Dodd, S.W., Pantoliano, M.W., Milenic, D.E., and Schlom, J. (1990). *In vivo* tumor targeting of a recombinant single-chain antigen-binding protein. *J. Natl. Cancer Inst.* **82**, 1191–1197.

156. Shimba, N., Torigoe, H., Takahashi, H., Masuda, K., Shimada, I., Arata, Y., and Sarai, A. (1995). Comparative thermodynamic analyses of the Fv, Fab* and Fab fragments of anti-dansyl mouse monoclonal antibody. *FEBS Lett.* **360**, 247–250.

157. Jung, S., and Pluckthun, A. (1997). Improving *in vivo* folding and stability of a single-chain Fv antibody fragment by loop grafting. *Protein Eng.* **10**, 959–966.

158. Proba, K., Worn, A., Honegger, A., and Pluckthun, A. (1998). Antibody scFv fragments without disulfide bonds made by molecular evolution. *J. Mol. Biol.* **275**, 245–253.

159. Marasco, W. (1997). *Intrabodies: from antibody genes to intracellular immunization*, Harwood academic, Amsterdam, NL.

160. Biocca, S., Pierandreu-Amaldi, P., and Cattaneo, A. (1993). Intracellular expression of anti-p21ras single chain Fv fragments inhibits meiotic maturation of *Xenopus* oocytes. *Biochem. Biophys. Res Commun.* **197**, 422–427.

161. Cardinale, A., Lener, M., Messina, S., Cattaneo, A., and Biocca, S. (1998). The mode of action of Y13–259 scFv fragment intracellularly expressed in mammalian cells. *FEBS Lett.* **439**, 197–202.

162. Cochet, O., Kenigsberg, M., Delumeau, I., Virone-Oddos, A., Multon, M., Fridman, W.H., Schweighoffer, F., Teillaud, J., and Tocqué, B. (1998). Intracellular expression of an antibody fragment-neutralizing p21 ras promotes tumor regression. *Cancer Res.* **58**, 1170–1176.

163. Marasco, W., Haseltine, W., and Chen, S. (1993). Design, intracellular expression, and activity of a human anti-human immunodeficiency virus type 1 gp 120 single-chain antibody, *Proc. Natl. Acad. Sci. USA* **90**, 7889–7893.

164. Zhou, P., Goldstein, S., Devadas, K., Tewari, D., and Notkins, A. L. (1998). Cells transfected with a non-neutralizing antibody gene are resistant to HIV infection: targeting the endoplasmic reticulum and trans-Golgi network. *J. Immunol.* **160**, 1489–1496.

165. Tewari, D., Goldstein, S.L., Notkins, A.L., and Zhou, P. (1998). cDNA encoding a single-chain antibody to HIV p17 with cytoplasmic or nuclear retention signals inhibits HIV-1 replication. *J. Immunol.* **161**, 2642–2647.

166. Caron de Fromentel, C., Gruel, N., Venot, C., Debussche, L., Conseiller, E., Dureuil, C., Teillaud, J. L., Tocque, B., and Bracco, L. (1999). Restoration of transcriptional activity of p53 mutants in human tumour cells by intracellular expression of anti-p53 single chain Fv fragments. *Oncogene* **18**, 551–557.

167. Mary, M.N., Venot, C., Caron de Fromentel, C., Debussche, L., Conseiller, E., Cochet, O., Gruel, N., Teillaud, J. L., Schweighoffer, F., Tocque, B., and Bracco, L. (1999). A tumor specific single chain antibody dependent gene expression system. *Oncogene* **18**, 559–564.

168. Smith, G.P. (1985). Filamentous fusion phage: novel expression vectors that display cloned antigens on the virion surface. *Science* **228**, 1315–1317.

169. Stahl, S., and Uhlen, M. (1997). Bacterial surface display: trends and progress. *Trends Biotechnol.* **15**, 185–192.

170. Kasahara, N., Dozy, A.M., and Kan, Y.W. (1994). Tissue–specific targeting of retroviral vectors through ligand–receptor interactions. *Science* **266**, 1373–1376.

171. Mattheakis, L.C., Bhatt, R.R., and Dower, W.J. (1994). An *in vitro* polysome display system for identifying ligands from very large peptide libraries. *Proc. Natl. Acad. Sci. USA* **91**, 9022–9026.

172. High, S., Gorlich, D., Wiedmann, M., Rapoport, T.A., and Dobberstein, B. (1991). The identification of proteins in the proximity of signal-anchor sequences during their targeting to and insertion into the membrane of the ER. *J. Cell Biol.* **113**, 35–44.

173. Fedorov, A.N., and Baldwin, T.O. (1995). Contribution of cotranslational folding to the rate of formation of native protein structure. *Proc. Natl. Acad. Sci. USA* **92**, 1227–1231.

174. Dower, W.J., Miller, J.F., and Ragsdale, C.W. (1988). High efficiency transformation of *E. coli* by high voltage electroporation. *Nucleic Acids Res.* **16**, 6127–6145.

175. Hanes, J., and Pluckthun, A. (1997). *In vitro* selection and evolution of functional proteins by using ribosome display. *Proc. Natl. Acad. Sci. USA* **94**, 4937–4942.

176. Ryabova, L.A., Desplancq, D., Spirin, A.S., and Pluckthun, A. (1997). Functional antibody production using cell-free translation: effects of protein disulfide isomerase and chaperones. *Nat. Biotechnol.* **15**, 79–84.

177. Hanes, J., Jermutus, L., Weber-Bornhauser, S., Bosshard, H.R., and Pluckthun, A. (1998). Ribosome display efficiently selects and evolves high-affinity antibodies *in vitro* from immune libraries. *Proc. Natl. Acad. Sci. USA* **95**, 14130–14135.

178. He, M., and Taussig, M.J. (1997). Antibody–ribosome–mRNA (ARM) complexes as efficient selection particles for *in vitro* display and evolution of antibody combining sites. *Nucleic Acids Res.* **25**, 5132–5134.

179. Roberts, R.W., and Szostak, J.W. (1997). RNA-peptide fusions for the *in vitro* selection of peptides and proteins. *Proc. Natl. Acad. Sci. USA* **94**, 12297–12302.

180. Nemoto, N., Miyamoto-Sato, E., Husimi, Y., and Yanagawa, H. (1997). *In vitro* virus: bonding of mRNA bearing puromycin at the 3′-terminal end to the C-terminal end of its encoded protein on the ribosome *in vitro*. *FEBS Lett.* **414**, 405–408.

181. Tawfik, D.S., and Griffiths, A.D. (1998). Man-made cell-like compartments for molecular evolution. *Nat. Biotechnol.* **16**, 652–656.

182. Better, M., Chang, C.P., Robinson, R.R., and Horwitz, A.H. (1988). *Escherichia coli* secretion of an active chimeric antibody fragment. *Science* **240**, 1041–1043.

183. Skerra, A., and Plückthun, A. (1988). Assembly of functional immunoglobulin Fv fragment in *Escherichia coli*. *Science* **240**, 1038–1040.

184. Wu, X.C., Ng, S.C., Near, R.I., and Wong, S.L. (1993). Efficient production of a functional single-chain antidigoxin antibody via an engineered *Bacillus subtilis* expression-secretion system. *Biotechnology* (NY). **11**, 71–76.

185. Horwitz, A.H., Chang, C.P., Better, M., Hellstrom, K.E., and Robinson, R.R. (1988). Secretion of functional antibody and Fab fragment from yeast cells. *Proc. Natl. Acad. Sci. USA* **85**, 8678–8682.

186. Edqvist, J., Keranen, S., Penttila, M., Straby, K.B., and Knowles, J.K. (1991). Production of functional IgM Fab fragments by *Saccharomyces cerevisiae*. *J. Biotechnol.* **20**, 291–300.

187. Bowdish, K., Tang, Y., Hicks, J.B., and Hilvert, D. (1991). Yeast expression of a catalytic antibody with chorismate mutase activity. *J. Biol. Chem.* **266**, 11901–11908.

188. Luo, D., Mah, N., Wishart, D., Zhang, Y., Jacobs, F., and Martin, L. (1996). Construction and expression of bi-functional proteins of single-chain Fv with effector domains. *J. Biochem (Tokyo).* **120**, 229–232.

189. Nyyssonen, E., Penttila, M., Harkki, A., Saloheimo, A., Knowles, J.K., and Keranen, S. (1993). Efficient production of antibody fragments by the filamentous fungus *Trichoderma reesei*. *Biotechnology* (N Y). **11**, 591–595.

190. Hsu, T.A., Eiden, J.J., and Betenbaugh, M.J. (1994). Engineering the assembly pathway of the baculovirus-insect cell expression system. *Ann. NY Acad. Sci.* **721**, 208–217.

191. Kretzschmar, T., Aoustin, L., Zingel, O., Marangi, M., Vonach, B., Towbin, H., and Geiser, M. (1996). High-level expression in insect cells and purification of secreted monomeric single-chain Fv antibodies. *J. Immunol. Meth.* **195**, 93–101.

192. Ward, V.K., Kreissig, S.B., Hammock, B.D., and Choudary, P.V. (1995). Generation of an expression library in the baculovirus expression vector system. *J. Virol. Methods.* **53**, 263–272.

193. Potter, K.N., Li, Z., and Capra, J.D. (1993). Antibody production in the baculovirus expression system. *Intern. Rev. Immunol.* **10**, 103–112.

194. Casadei, J., Powell, M.J., and Kenten, J.H. (1990). Expression and secretion of aequorin as a chimeric antibody by means of a mammalian expression vector. *Proc. Natl. Acad. Sci. USA* **87**, 2047–2051.

195. Gilliland, L.K., Norris, N.A., Marquardt, H., Tsu, T.T., Hayden, M.S., Neubauer, M.G., Yelton, D.E., Mittler, R.S., and Ledbetter, J.A. (1996). Rapid and reliable cloning of antibody variable regions and generation of recombinant single chain antibody fragments. *Tissue Antigens* **47**, 1–20.

196. Jost, C.R., Kurucz, I., Jacobus, C.M., Titus, J.A., George, A.J.T., and Segal, D.M. (1994). Mammalian expression and secretion of functional single-chain Fv molecules. *J. Biol. Chem.* **269**, 26267–26273.

197. Hiatt, A., and Ma, J.K. (1993). Characterization and applications of antibodies produced in plants. *Int. Rev. Immunol.* **10**, 139–152.

198. Hiatt, A., and Mostov, K. (1992). Assembly of multimeric proteins in plant cells: characteristics and uses of plant-derived antibodies: in *Transgenic Plants: Fundamentals and Applications* (Hiatt, A., ed) pp. 221–236, Marcel Dekker Inc., New York.

199. Hiatt, A.C. (1991). Production of monoclonal antibody in plants. *Transplant Proc.* **23**, 147–151, discussion 151.

200. Hiatt, A. (1990). Antibodies produced in plants. *Nature* **344**, 469–470.

201. Conrad, U., Fiedler, U., Artsaenko, O., and Phillips, J. (1998). High level and stable accumulation of Single chain Fv antibodies in Plant Storage Organs. *J. Plant Physiol.* **152**, 708–711.

202. Conrad, U., and Fiedler, U. (1998). Compartment-specific accumulation of recombinant immunoglobulins in plant cells: an essential tool for antibody production and immunomodulation of physiological functions and pathogen activity. *Plant Mol. Biol.* **38**, 101–109.

203. Fischer, R., Drossard, J., Hellwig, S., Emans, N., and Schillberg, S. (1998). Transgenic plants as bioreactors for the expression of recombinant antibodies. in *Proceedings of the Xth International Congress of Immunology* (Talwar, N., ed) pp. 307–313, Monduzzi Editore Publishers, Bologna.

204. Fischer, R., Voss, A., Stierhof, Y.-D., and Kreuzaler, F. (*Submitted*) Production, characterisation and molecular cloning of Tobacco Mosaic Virus (TMV)-specific neutralizing monoclonal antibodies with different epitope specificities, *Mol. Immunol.*

205. Fischer, R., Drossard, J., Liao, Y.C., and Schillberg, S. (1998). Characterisation and applications of plant-derived recombinant antibodies in *Methods in biotechnology Vol. 3: Recombinant proteins in plants: Production and Isolation of Clinically useful compounds.* (Cunningham, C., and Porter, A. J. R., eds), Humana Press, Totowa, NJ.

206. Huston, J.S., Mudgett-Hunter, M., Tai, M.-S., McCartney, J., Warren, F., Haber, E., and Oppermann, H. (1991). Protein engineering of single-chain Fv analogs and fusion proteins in *Methods in Enzymology* pp. 46–88, Academic Press.

207. Buchner, J., Brinkmann, U., and Pastan, I. (1992). Renaturation of a single-chain immunotoxin facilitated by chaperones and protein disulphide isomerase. *Biotechnology* **10**, 682–685.

208. Buchner, J., Pastan, I., and Brinkmann, U. (1992). A method for increasing the yield of properly folded recombinant fusion proteins: Single-chain immunotoxin from renaturation of bacterial inclusion bodies. *Anal. Biochem.* **205**, 263–270.

209. Buchner, J., and Rudolph, R. (1991). Renaturation, purification and characterization of recombinant Fab-fragments produced in E.coli. *Bio/Tech.* **9**, 157–162.

210. Freund, C., Ross, A., Plueckthun, A., and Holak, T.A. (1994). Structural and dynamic properties of the Fv fragment and the single-chain Fv fragment of an antibody in solution investigated by heteronuclear three-dimensional NMR spectroscopy. *Biochem.* **33**, 3296–3303.

211. Skerra, A., Pfitzinger, I., and Plückthun, A. (1991). The functional expression of antibody Fv fragments in *Escherichia coli:* improved vectors and a generally applicable purification technique. *Bio/Tech.* **9**, 273–278.

212. Skerra, A., and Plueckthun, A. (1991). Secretion and *in vivo* folding of the Fab fragment of the antibody McPC603 in *Escherichia coli:* influence of disulphides and cis-prolines. *Protein Engineering* **4**, 971–979.

213. Anthony, J., Near, R., Wong, S.L., Iida, E., Ernst, E., Wittekind, M., Haber, E., and Ng, S.C. (1992). Production of stable anti-digoxin Fv in *Escherichia coli, Mol. Immunol.* **29**, 1237–1247.

214. Pluckthun, A., and Skerra, A. (1989). Expression of functional antibody Fv and Fab fragments in *Escherichia coli. Methods Enzymol.* **178**, 497–515.

215. Froyen, G., Ronsse, I., and Billiau, A. (1993). Bacterial expression of a single-chain antibody fragment (SCFV) that neutralizes the biological activity of human interferon-gamma. *Mol. Immunol.* **30**, 805–812.

216. Bejcek, B.E., Wang, D., Berven, E., Pennell, C.A., Peiper, S.C., Poppema, S., Uckun, F.M., and Kersey, J.H. (1995). Development and characterization of three recombinant single chain antibody fragments (scFvs) directed against the CD19 antigen. *Cancer Res.* **55**, 2346–2351.

217. Huston, J.S., Levinson, D., Mudgett, H.M., Tai, M.S., Novotny, J., Margolies, M.N., Ridge, R.J., Bruccoleri, R.E., Haber, E., Crea, R., and Opperman, H. (1988). Protein engineering of antibody binding sites: recovery of specific activity in an anti-digoxin single-chain Fv analogue produced in *Escherichia coli. Proc. Natl. Acad. Sci. USA* **85**, 5879–5883.

218. Bird, R.E., Hardman, K.D., Jacobson, J.W., Johnson, S., Kaufman, B.M., Lee, S.M., Lee, T., Pope, S.H., Riordan, G.S., and Whitlow, M. (1988). Single-chain antigen-binding proteins [published erratum appears in Science 1989 Apr 28;244(4903):409]. *Science* **242**, 423–426.

219. Horn, U., Strittmatter, W., Krebber, A., Knupfer, U., Kujau, M., Wenderoth, R., Muller, K., Matzku, S., Pluckthun, A., and Riesenberg, D. (1996). High volumetric yields of functional dimeric miniantibodies in *Escherichia coli*, using an optimized expression vector and high-cell-density fermentation under non-limited growth conditions. *Applied Microbiology and Biotechnology.* **46**, 524–532.

220. Higgins, D.R., and Cregg, J.M. (1998). Introduction to *Pichia pastoris:* in *Pichia Protocols* (Higgins, D. R., and Cregg, J.M., eds) pp. 1–15, Humana Press, Totowa, NJ.

221. Sreekrishna, K., Brankamp, R.G., Kropp, K.E., Blankenship, D.T., Tsay, J.T., Smith, P.L., Wierschke, J.D., Subramaniam, A., and Birkenberger, L.A. (1997). Strategies for optimal synthesis and secretion of heterologous proteins in the methylotrophic yeast *Pichia pastoris. Gene* **190**, 55–62.

222. Cregg, J. (1999). Expression in the methylotrophic yeast *Pichia pastoris* in *Gene expression systems: Using nature for the art of expression* (Fernandez, J., and Hoeffler, J., eds) pp. 158–184, Academic Press, San Diego, CA.

223. Pichuantes, S., Nguyen, A., and Franzusoff, A. (1996). *Expression of heterologus gene products in yeast*, Wiley Liss, New York.

224. Hollenberg, C.P., and Gellissen, G. (1997). Production of recombinant proteins by methylotrophic yeasts. *Curr. Opin. Biotechnol.* **8**, 554–560.

225. Canales, M., Enriquez, A., Ramos, E., Cabrera, D., Dandie, H., Soto, A., Falcon, V., Rodriguez, M., and de la Fuente, J. (1997). Large-scale production in *Pichia pastoris* of the recombinant vaccine Gavac against cattle tick. *Vaccine* **15**, 414–422.

226. O'Donohue, M.J., Boissy, G., Huet, J.C., Nespoulous, C., Brunie, S., and Pernollet, J.C. (1996). Overexpression in *Pichia pastoris* and crystallization of an elicitor protein secreted by the phytopathogenic fungus, *Phytophthora cryptogea*. *Protein Expr. Purif.* **8**, 254–261.

227. Fischer, M., Goldschmitt, J., Peschel, C., Brakenhoff, J.P., Kallen, K.J., Wollmer, A., Grotzinger, J., and Rose-John, S. (1997). I. A bioactive designer cytokine for human hematopoietic progenitor cell expansion. *Nat. Biotechnol.* **15**, 142–145.

228. Taticek, R.A., Lee, C.W.T., and Shukler, M.L. (1994). *Curr. Opin. Biotech.* **5**, 165–174.

229. Skerra, A. (1993). *Curr. Opin. Biotech.* **5**, 165–714.

230. Echelard, Y. (1996). Recombinant protein production in transgenic animals. *Curr. Opin. Biotechnol.* **7**, 536–540.

231. Gorman, C.M. (1990). Mammalian cell expression. *Curr. Opin. Biotechnol.* **1**, 36–47.

232. Potrykus, I. (1991). *Annu. Rev. Plant Physiol. Plant Mol. Biol.* **42**, 205–225.

233. Ma, J., and Hein, M. (1995). Immunotherpeuic potential of antibodies produced in plants. *Trends Biotechnol.* **13**, 522–527.

234. Mason, H.S., and Arntzen, C.J. (1995). Transgenic plants as vaccine production systems. *Trends Biotechnol.* **13**, 388–392.

235. McCormick, A.A., Kumagai, M.H., Hanley, K., Turpen, T.H., Hakim, I., Grill, L.K., Tusé, D., Levy, S., and Levy, R. (1999). Rapid production of specific vaccines for lymphoma by expression of the tumor-derived single-chain Fv epitopes in tobacco plants. *Proc. Natl. Acad. Sci. USA.* **8**, 255–263.

236. Schillberg, S., Zimmermann, S., Voss, A., and Fischer, R. (1999). Apoplastic and cytosolic expression of full-size antibodies and antibody fragments in *Nicotiana tabacum*. *Transgenic Research* **8**, 255–263.

237. Schillberg, S., Zimmermann, S., Findlay, K., and Fischer, R. (2000). Plasma membrane display of antiviral single chain Fv fragments confers resistance to tobocco mosaic virus. *Molecular Breeding* **6**, 317–326

238. Fischer, R., Schumann, D., Zimmermann, S., Drossard, J., Sack, M., and Schillberg, S. (1999) Expression and characterization of bispecific single chain Fv fragments produced in transgenic plants. *European J. Biochemistry* **262**, 810–816

239. Zimmermann, S., Schillberg, S., Liao, Y.C., and Fischer, R. (1998). Intracellular expression of TMV-specific single-chain Fv fragments leads to improved virus resistance in *Nicotiana tabacum*. *Molecular Breeding* **4**, 369–379.

240. Tavladoraki, P., Benvenuto, E., Trinca, S., De Martinis, D., Cattaneo, A., and Galeffi, P. (1993). Transgenic plants expressing a functional single-chain Fv antibody are specifically protected from virus attack. *Nature* **366**, 469–472.

241. Firek, S., Draper, J., Owen, M.R., Gandecha, A., Cockburn, B., and Whitelam, G.C. (1993). Secretion of a functional single-chain Fv protein in transgenic tobacco plants and cell suspension cultures [published erratum appears in *Plant Mol. Biol. 1994* Mar.; **24(5)**: 833]. *Plant Mol. Biol.* **23**, 861–870.

242. De Wilde, C., De Rycke, R., Beeckman, T., De Neve, M., Van Montagu, M., Engler, G., and Depicker, A. (1998). Accumulation pattern of IgG antibodies and Fab fragments in transgenic Arabidopsis thaliana plants. *Plant Cell Physiol.* **39**, 639–646.

243. De Jaeger, G., Buys, E., Eeckhout, D., De Wilde, C., Jacobs, A., Kapila, J., Angenon, G., Van Montagu, M., Gerats, T., and Depicker, A. (1998). High level accumulation of single-chain variable fragments in the cytosol of transgenic *Petunia hybrida*. *Eur. J. Biochem.* **259**, 1–10.

244. Artsaenko, O., Kettig, B., Fiedler, U., Conrad, U., and Düring, K. (1998). Potato tubers as a biofactory for recombinant antibodies. *Mol. Breeding* **4**, 313–319.

245. Voloudakis, A., Yin, Y., and Beachy, R. (1999). Recombinant protein expression in plants in *Gene expression systems: Using nature for the art of expression* (Fernandez, J., and Hoeffler, J., eds) pp. 429–461, Academic Press, San Diego, CA.

246. Christou, P. (1993). Particle gun-mediated transformation. *Current Opinion in Biotechnology* **4**, 135–141.

247. Kapila, J., De Rycke, R., van Montagu, M., and Angenon, G. (1996). An *Agrobacterium* mediated transient gene expression system for intact leaves. *Plant Sci.* **122**, 101–108.

248. Verch, T., Yusibov, V., and Koprowski, H. (1998). Expression and assembly of a full-length monoclonal antibody in plants using a plant virus vector. *J. Immunol. Meth.* **220**, 69–75.

249. Smolenska, L., Robert, I., Learmouth, H., Porter, A., Harris, W., Wilson, T., and Santa Cruz, S. (1998). Production of a functional single chain antibody attached to the surface of a plant virus. *FEBS lett.* **441**, 379–382.

250. Hiatt, A., Tang, Y., Weiser, W., and Hein, M.B. (1992). Assembly of antibodies and mutagenized variants in transgenic plants and plant cell cultures, *Genet Eng.* **14**, 49–64.

251. Kusnadi, A.R., Nikolov, Z.L., and Howard, J.A. (1997). Production of recombinant proteins in transgenic plants: Practical Considerations. *Biotechnol. Bioeng.* **56**, 473–484.

252. Baum, T.J., Hiatt, A., Parrott, W.A., Pratt, L.H., and Hussey, R.S. (1996). Expression in tobacco of a functional monoclonal antibody specific to stylet secretions of the root-knot nematode. *MPMI.* **9**, 382–387.

253. De Wilde, C., De Neve, M., De Rycke, R., Bruyns, A.M., De Jaeger, G., Van Montagu, M., Depicker, A., and Engler, G. (1996). Intact antigen-binding MAK33 antibody and Fab fragment accumulate in intercellular spaces of *Arabidopsis thaliana. Plant Science* **114**, 233–241.

254. Voss, A., Niersbach, M., Hain, R., Hirsch, H., Liao, Y., Kreuzaler, F., and Fischer, R. (1995). Reduced virus infectivity in *N. tabacum* secreting a TMV-specific full size antibody. *Mol. Breeding.* **1**, 39–50.

255. Ma, J.K.C., Lehner, T., Stabila, P., Fux, C. I., and Hiatt, A. (1994). Assembly of monoclonal antibodies with IgG1 and IgA heavy chain domains in transgenic tobacco plants. *Eur. J. Immunol.* **24**, 131–138.

256. De Neve, M., De Loose, M., Jacobs, A., Van Houdt, H., Kaluza, B., Weidle, U., Van Montagu, M., and Depicker, A. (1993). Assembly of an antibody and its derived antibody fragment in *Nicotiana* and *Arabidopsis. Transgenic Res.* **2**, 227–237.

257. Artsaenko, O., Peisker, M., zur Nieden, U., Fiedler, U., Weiler, E.W., Müntz, K., and Conrad, U. (1995). Expression of a single-chain Fv antibody against abscisic acid creates a wilty phenotype in transgenic tobacco. *The Plant J.* **8**, 745–750.

258. Fiedler, U., and Conrad, U. (1995). High-level production and long-term storage of engineered antibodies in transgenic tobacco seeds. *Bio/Tech.* **13**, 1090–1093.

259. Fiedler, U., Philips, J., Artsaenko, O., and Conrad, U. (1997). Optimisation of scFv antibody production in transgenic plants. *Immunotechnology* **3**, 205–216.

260. Owen, M., Gandecha, A., Cockburn, B., and Whitelam, G. (1992). Synthesis of a functional anti-phytochrome single-chain Fv protein in transgenic tobacco. *Biotechnology* (N Y). **10**, 790–794.

261. Schouten, A., Roosien, J., van Engelen, F.A., de Jong, G.A.M., Borst-Vrenssen, A.W.M., Zilverentant, J.F., Bosch, D., Stiekema, W.J., Gommers, F.J., Schots, A., and Bakker, J. (1996). The C-terminal KDEL sequence increases the expression level of a single-chain antibody designed to be targeted to both cytosol and the secretory pathway in transgenic tobacco. *Plant Mol. Biol.* **30**, 781–793.

262. Schouten, A., Roosien, J., de Boer, J.M., Wilmink, A., Rosso, M.N., Bosch, D., Stiekema, W.J., Gommers, F.J., Bakker, J., and Schots, A. (1997). Improving scFv antibody expression levels in the plant cytosol. *FEBS Lett.* **415**, 235–241.

263. van Engelen, F.A., Schouten, A., Molthoff, J.W., Roosien, J., Salinas, J., Dirkse, W.G., Schots, A., Bakker, J., Gommers, F.J., Jongsma, M.A., and *et al.* (1994). Coordinate expression of antibody subunit genes yields high levels of functional antibodies in roots of transgenic tobacco. *Plant Mol. Biol.* **26**, 1701–1710.

264. Ma, J.K., Hiatt, A., Hein, M., Vine, N.D., Wang, F., Stabila, P., van Dolleweerd, C., Mostov, K., and Lehner, T. (1995). Generation and assembly of secretory antibodies in plants. *Science* **268**, 716–719.

265. Phillips, J., Artsaencko, O., Fiedler, U., Horstmann, C., Mock, H.P., Müntz, K., and Conrad, U. (1997). Seed-specific immunomodulation of abscisic acid activity induces a developmental switch. *EMBO.* **16**, 4489–4496.

266. Taticek, R.A., Lee, C.W.T., and Shuler, M. L. (1994). Large-scale insect and plant cell culture. *Curr. Opin. Biotechnol.* **5**, 165–174.

267. Scragg, A.H. (1992). Large-scale plant cell culture: methods, applications and products. *Curr. Opin. Biotechnol.* **3**, 105–109.

268. Drossard, J., Liao, Y.-C., and Fischer, R. (1999). Affinity-purification of a TMV-specific recombinant full-size antibody from a transgenic tobacco suspension culture. *J. Immunol. Meth.* **266**, 1–10

269. Francisco, J.A., Gawlak, S.L., Miller, M., Bathe, J., Russell, D., Chace, D., Mixan, B., Zhao, L., Fell, H.P., and Siegall, C.B. (1997). Expression and characterization of bryodin 1 and a bryodin 1-based single-chain immunotoxin from tobacco cell culture. *Bioconjug. Chem.* **8**, 708–713.

270. Gallie, D. (1998). Controlling gene expression in transgenics. *Curr. Opin. Plant Biol.* **1**, 166–172.

271. Blobel, G., and Dobberstein, B. (1975). Transfer of proteins across membranes I. Presence of proteolytically processed and unprocessed nascent immunoglobulin light chains on membrane-bound ribosomes of murine myeloma. *J. Cell Biol.* **67**, 835–851.

272. Denecke, J., Goldman, M.H.S., Demolder, J., Seurinck, J., and Botterman, J. (1991). The tobacco luminal binding protein is encoded by a multigene family. *Plant Cell* **3**, 1025–1035.

273. Baker, D., and Harkonen, W. (1990). Regulatory agency concerns in the manufacturing and testing of monoclonal antibodies for therapeutic use. *Targeted Diagn. Ther.* **3**, 75–98.

274. Mariani, M., and Tarditi, L. (1992). Validating the preparation of clinical monoclonal antibodies. *Biotechnology* **10**, 394–396.

275. Murano, G. (1997). FDA perspective on specifications for biotechnology products–from IND to PLA. *Dev. Biol. Stand.* **91**, 3–13.

276. Miele, L. (1997). *Tibech.* **15**, 45–50.

277. Moloney, M.M., and Holbrook, L.A. (1997). Subcellular targeting and purification of recombinant proteins in plant production systems. *Biotechnol. Genet. Eng. Rev.* **14**, 321–36.

278. van Regenmortel, M.H.V. (1986). Tobacco Mosaic Virus: Antigenic Structure in *Plant Viruses*, **Vol 2** pp. 79–104, Plenum Press, New York.

279. Cabanes-Macheteau, M., Fitchette-lainé, A.-C., Loutelier-Bourhis, C., Lange, C., Ma, J., Lerouge, P., and Faye, L. (1999). N–glycosylation of a mouse IgG expressed in transgenic tobacco plants. *Glycobiology* **9**, 365–372.

280. Longstaff, M., Newell, C.A., Boonstra, B., Strachan, G., Learmonth, D., Harris, W.J., Porter, A.J., and Hamilton, W.D. (1998). Expression and characterisation of single-chain antibody fragments produced in transgenic plants against the organic herbicides atrazine and paraquat. *Biochimica Et Biophysica Acta.* **1381**, 147–160.

281. Biocca, S., and Cattaneo, A. (1995). Intracellular immunization: antibody targeting to subcellular compartments. *Trends in Cell Biology* **5**, 248–252.

282. Richardson, J.H., and Marasco, W.A. (1995). Intracellular antibodies: development and therapeutic potential. *TIBTECH* **13**, 306–310.

283. Cattaneo, A., and Biocca, S. (1999). The selection of intracellular antibodies. *Trends in Biotechnology* **17**, 115–121.

284. Takata, R., Miyamoto, Y., Honjoh, K., Soeda, T., Sakamoto, J., Miyamoto, T., and Hatano, S. (1998). Antibody fragments as inhibitors of Japanese radish acid phosphatase. *Biosci. Biotechnol. Biochem.* **62**, 1041–1047.

285. Le Gall, F., Bove, J.M., and Garnier, M. (1998). Engineering of a single-chain variable-fragment (scFv) antibody specific for the stolbur phytoplasma (Mollicute) and its expression in *Escherichia coli* and tobacco plants. *Applied Environmental Microbiology* **64**, 4566–4572.

286. Fecker, L. F., Koenig, R., and Obermeier, C. (1997). Nicotiana benthamiana plants expressing beet necrotic yellow vein virus (BNYVV) coat protein-specific scFv are partially protected against the establishment of the virus in the early stages of infection and its pathogenic effects in the late stages of infection. *Arch Virol.* **142**, 1857–1863.

287. Lomonossoff, G.P. (1995). Pathogen-derived resistance to plant viruses. *Annu. Rev. Phytopathol.* **33**, 323–343.

288. Dawson, W.O. (1996). Gene silencing and virus resistance: a common mechanism. *Trends Plant Sci.* **1**, 107–108.

289. Lam, Y.H., Wong, Y.S., Wang, B., Wong, R.N.S., Yeung, H.W., and Shaw, P.C. (1996). Use of trichosanthin to reduce infection by turnip mosaic virus. *Plant Science* **114**, 111–117.

290. Taylor, S., Massiah, A., Lomonossoff, G., Roberts, L.M., Lord, J.M., and Hartley, M. (1994). Correlation between the activities of five ribosome-inactivating proteins in depurination of tobacco ribosomes and inhibition of tobacco mosaic virus infection. *Plant J.* **5**, 827–835.

291. Lin, W., Anuratha, C.S., Datta, K., Potrykus, I., Mathukrishnan, S., and Datta, S.K. (1995). Genetic engineering of rice for resistance to sheath blight. *BioTechnology* **13**, 686–691.

292. Masoud, S.A., Zhu, Q., Lamb, C., and Dixon, R.A. (1996). Constitutive expression of an inducible beta-1,3-glucanase in alfalfa reduces disease severity caused by the oomycete pathogen *Phytophtora megasperma* f-sp. *medicagini*, but does not reduce disease severity of chitin-containing fungi. *Transgenic Research* **5**, 313–323.

293. Marasco, W.A. (1995). Intracellular antibodies (intrabodies) as research reagents and therapeutic molecules for gene therapy. *Immunotechnology* **1**, 1–19.

294. Baulcombe, D. (1994). Novel strategies for engineering virus resistance in plants. *Curr. Opin. Biotechnol.* **5**, 117–124.

295. Wilson, T. (1993). Strategies to protect crop plants against viruses: Pathogen-derived resistance blossoms. *Proc. Natl. Acad. Sci. USA* **90**, 3134–3141.

296. Ma, J.K., Hiatt, A., Hein, M., Vine, N.D., Wang, F., Stabila, P., van Dolleweerd, C., Mostov, K., and Lehner, T. (1995). Generation and assembly of secretory antibodies in plants. *Science* **268**, 716–719.

297. Mostov, K.E. (1994). Transepithelial transport of immunoglobulins. *Annu. Rev. Immunol.* **12**, 63–84.

298. Ahnen, D.J., Singleton, J.R., Hoops, T.C., and Kloppel, T.M. (1986). Posttranslational processing of secretory component in the rat jejunum by a brush border metalloprotease. *J. Clin. Invest.* **77**, 1841–1848.

299. Zeitlin, L., Cone, R.A., and Whaley, K.J. (1999). Using Monoclonal Antibodies to Prevent Mucosal Transmission of Epidemic Infectious Diseases. *Emerging Infectious Diseases* **5**, 54–64.

300. Lehner, T., Caldwell, J., and Smith, R. (1985). Local passive immunization by monoclonal antibodies against streptococcal antigen I/II in the prevention of dental caries. *Infect. Immun.* **50**, 796–799.

301. Loesche, W.J. (1986). Role of *Streptococcus mutans* in human dental decay. *Microbiol Rev.* **50**, 353–380.

302. Underdown, B.J., and Dorrington, K.J. (1974). Studies on the structural and conformational basis for the relative resistance of serum and secretory immunoglobulin A to proteolysis. *J. Immunol.* **112**, 949–959.
303. Kraehenbuhl, J.P., and Neutra, M.R. (1992). Molecular and cellular basis of immune protection of mucosal surfaces. *Physiol. Rev.* **1992**, 853–879.
304. Winner, L.d., Mack, J., Weltzin, R., Mekalanos, J.J., Kraehenbuhl, J.P., and Neutra, M.R. (1991). New model for analysis of mucosal immunity: intestinal secretion of specific monoclonal immunoglobulin A from hybridoma tumors protects against *Vibrio cholerae* infection. *Infect. Immun.* **59**, 977–982.
305. Chintalacharuvu, K.R., and Morrison, S.L. (1997). Production of secretory immunoglobulin A by a single mammalian cell. *Proc. Natl. Acad. Sci. USA* **94**, 6364–6368.
306. Michalek, S.M., Gregory, R.L., Harmon, C.C., Katz, J., Richardson, G.J., Hilton, T., Filler, S.J., and McGhee, J.R. (1987). Protection of gnotobiotic rats against dental caries by passive immunization with bovine milk antibodies to *Streptococcus mutans*. *Infect. Immun.* **55**, 2341–2347.
307. Komari, T., Hiei, Y., Ishida, Y., Kumashiro, T., and Kubo, T. (1998). Advances in cereal gene transfer. *Curr. Opin. Plant Biol.* **1**, 161–165.
308. Wassenegger, M., and Pelissier, T. (1998). A model for RNA-mediated gene silencing in higher plants. *Plant Mol. Biol.* **37**, 349–362.
309. Verwoerd, T.C., van Paridon, P.A., van Ooyen, A.J.J., van Lent, J.W.M., Hoekema, A., and Pen, J. (1995). *Plant Physiol.* **109**, 1199–1205.
310. Larrick, J.W., Yu, L., Chen, J., Jaiswal, S., and Wycoff, K. (1998). Production of antibodies in transgenic plants [In Process Citation]. *Res. Immunol.* **149**, 603–608.
311. Köhler, G., and Milstein, C. (1975). Continuous cultures of fused cells secreting antibody of predefined specificit. *Nature* **256**, 495–497.
312. Goldenberg, D.M., DeLand, F., Kim, E., Bennett, S., Primus, F. J., van Nagell J.R. Jr., Estes, N., DeSimone, P., and Rayburn, P. (1978). Use of radiolabeled antibodies to carcinoembryonic antigen for the detection and localization of diverse cancers by external photoscanning. *New England Journal Of Medicine* **298**, 1384–1386.
313. Miller, R.A., Maloney, D.G., Warnke, R., and Levy, R. (1982). Treatment of B-cell lymphoma with monoclonal anti-idiotype antibody. *New England Journal of Medicine* **306**, 517–522.
314. Boss, J.M., and Strominger, J.L. (1984). Cloning and sequence analysis of the human major histocompatibility complex gene DC-3 beta. *Proc. Natl. Acad. Sci. USA* **81**, 5199–5203.
315. Cabilly, S., Riggs, A.D., Pande, H., Shively, J.E., Holmes, W.E., Michael, R., Perry, L.J., Wetzel, R., and Heynecker, H.L. (1984). Generation of antibody activity from immunoglobulin and polypeptide chains produced in *E. coli*. *Proc. Natl. Acad. Sci. USA* **81**, 3273–3277.
316. Spitler, L.E., del Rio, M., Khentigan, A., Wedel, N.I., Brophy, N.A., Miller, L.L., Harkonen, W.S., Rosendorf, L.L., Lee, H.M., Mischak, R.P., and et a (1987). Therapy of patients with malignant melanoma using a monoclonal antimelanoma antibody-ricin A chain immunotoxin. *Cancer Research*. **47**, 1717–1723.
317. Minagawa, H., Sakuma, S., Mohri, S., Mori, R., and Watanabe, T. (1988). *Herpes simplex* virus type 1 infection in mice with severe combined immunodeficiency (SCID). *Archives of Virology*. **103**, 73–82.
318. Mathieson, P.W., Cobbold, S.P., Hale, G., Clark, M.R., Oliveira, D.B., Lockwood, C.M., and Waldmann, H. (1990). Monoclonal-antibody therapy in systemic vasculitis. *N. Engl. J. Med.* **323**, 250–254.
319. Benvenuto, E., Ordas, R.J., Tavazza, R., Ancora, G., Biocca, S., Cattaneo, A., and Galeffi, P. (1991). "Phytoantibodies": a general vector for the expression of immunoglobulin domains in transgenic plants. *Plant Mol. Biol.* **17**, 865–874.

320. Fecker, L.F., Kaufmann, A., Commandeur, U., Commandeur, J., Koenig, R., and Burgermeister, W. (1996). Expression of single-chain antibody fragments (scFv) specific for beet necrotic yellow vein virus coat protein or 25kDa protein in *Escherichia coli* and *Nicotiana benthamiana*. *Plant Mol. Biol.* **32**, 979–986.
321. Bruyns, A.M., De Jaeger, G., De Neve, M., De Wilde, C., Van Montagu, M., and Depicker, A. (1996). Bacterial and plant-produced scFv proteins have similar antigen-binding properties. *FEBS Letters* **386**, 5–10.
322. Ridder, R., and al., e. (1995). Generation of rabbit monoclonal antbody fragments from a combinatorial phage display library and their production in the yeast *Pichia pastoris*. *Bio/Tech.* **13**, 255–260.
323. Eldin, P., Pauza, M.E., Hieda, Y., Lin, G., Murtaugh, M.P., Pentel, P.R., and Pennell, C.A. (1997). High-level secretion of two antibody single chain Fv fragments by *Pichia pastoris*. *J. Immunol. Methods* **201**, 67–75.

INDEX: Volume 7

INDEX: Volumes 1–6

171

D

CONTENTS OF PREVIOUS VOLUMES

Printed and bound by CPI Group (UK) Ltd, Croydon, CR0 4YY

23/10/2024

01778226-0003